THE WHOLE TRUTH

ABOUT BEAUTY, YOUTH, AND SKINCARE

A former beautician from Los Angeles finally reveals the true secrets
of beautiful, healthy, and glowing skin that any woman can attain
without expensive cosmetic procedures or plastic surgery!

RUTA BANIONYTE

The information in this book is for educational purposes only. It is not meant to diagnose or treat skin problems. In this book, I share my knowledge and experience related to skin care, beauty, and nutrition. Please contact your doctor for specific skin, weight, or psychological problems and appropriate treatment.

The truth is that for half of my life, I couldn't accept the way I looked. Breakouts, brown spots, enlarged pores, wrinkles and fine lines, dull complexion, and drooping eyelids were my reality, annoying and destroying my self-esteem.

I remember looking in the mirror and bursting into tears in desperation over enormous cystic acne. I cannot forget feeling miserable over an early appearance of fine lines. My skin condition was so poor, I couldn't face myself or anyone else in broad daylight.

I paid numerous visits to dermatologists, nutritionists, and other types of "-ists" in Europe and Los Angeles, USA. I tried different creams, hormone therapy, antibiotics, and a variety of diets. I spent a small fortune on all of that, but the desired results never came. A miracle solution—pill, ointment, cream—seemed to be right in front of me only to end up, yet again, to be a disappointing waste of time a few weeks later. I was beginning to lose hope that the situation would improve.

In complete despair, I finally realized that the only way to help myself was to *become a beautician* and to learn what was happening to my body and my skin. So I enrolled in a beauty school in Los Angeles and immersed myself in an intensive search for the answers.

The road to uncovering the true beauty secrets (not the obvious lies the cosmetic industry feeds us every day) was long and painful. The lack of knowledge was at the root of my problems.

In sunny California, I was learning beauty secrets from the best teachers at the time (including Janel Luu, the founder of famous "LE MIEUX" cosmetic products). I graduated from the National Academy of Sports Medicine, successfully operating in the USA since 1987. After obtaining the cosmetology license in California, I started working in beauty salons in Los Angeles.

Staying in this field for a long time was not my plan. The only goal of becoming a beautician was to help MYSELF. The way I see beauty now was largely influenced by an 80-something-year-old lady, an instructor from Thailand. She generously shared many secrets from the East where women start taking care of their skin very early and protect it for the rest of their lives. As soon as I started to uncover beauty secrets, my life started to change. For the next several years, I gained necessary knowledge about *feminine beauty and youth preservation.*

Over the course of my long studies and experimentation with my own problematic skin, I discovered *the main principles of skin care and beauty* and researched the effects of the food we eat. I learned to notice what *really* works and what is just an empty promise or false advertisement.

I also learned how fine lines and wrinkles appear, how to stay slim and beautiful for a long time, why diets don't work and how to replace them, why our skin ages, and how to slow down this process.

I will never know why the dermatologists, dietitians, and other beauticians wouldn't tell me the whole truth about beauty when I was younger. Maybe they were paid by Big Pharma and the giants of the cosmetics industry, or maybe they just did not know any better.

I wrote this book so that you don't have to learn this previously hidden information the hard way like I did. My goal is to give you real and valuable knowledge about skin care and how to preserve your beauty. You will find that the book is easy to read, easy to understand, and it can really change your life!

BUT FIRST, LET ME BRIEFLY
DESCRIBE THE JOURNEY
YOU ARE ABOUT TO TAKE.

IN CHAPTER ONE

I will give some insights about how women make themselves age prematurely without even knowing it. We will discuss negative beliefs about youth, beauty, and aging. Maybe you are asking yourself why, in the book about beauty and youth, we should talk about the topics more suitable for self-help and positive thinking?

I am convinced that self-improvement and positive beliefs are the basis of feminine beauty. A woman will never be beautiful, happy, and glowing if she holds on to too many beliefs that age her. Yes, in this book, we will talk a lot about skin care and effective products; however, if we don't pay attention to our beliefs, it will be really difficult to get good results.

Holding on to negative beliefs about beauty and youth is like throwing a wrench into your efforts. First, we have to remove that "wrench" in order to keep moving forward. In this chapter, we will discuss the main destructive beliefs about beauty and youth, and then we will look at 5 steps to deal with them.

IN CHAPTER TWO

I will openly share with you my constant disappointments and quests to solve my embarrassing skin problems. They started when I was fourteen. My face looked so catastrophic, it made me burst into tears every time I looked in the mirror. The worst thing was that as soon as I solved one skin problem, another one suddenly appeared. At first there was acne. Later, brown spots. After a while, fine lines, dull dry skin, dark circles under the eyes . . . It was never ending.

I couldn't understand what I was doing wrong until the start of my long-term studies about skin care and beauty. Let me tell you a secret: my greatest influence was a beautiful elderly lady from Thailand. But more about that later.

IN CHAPTER THREE

we'll talk about the beauty industry myths and white lies which caused me to waste tons of money and time! I'll be honest, writing this chapter was the most unpleasant. It makes me really sad when I think about the time and money spent on bogus advice and products. Given so much choice, it's almost impossible to know which products or procedures really work. After reading this chapter, you will feel like you have received a gift—you will finally know what is useful and effective in the cosmetics industry, and what is a simple lie not worth your attention. We'll discuss 27 beauty industry myths, including usefulness of undereye creams, effectiveness of natural products, expensive cosmetics, trendy supplements, tonics, homemade masks, cellulite, micellar water, and so much more! This chapter will definitely be helpful and thought-provoking.

CHAPTER FOUR

will be dedicated to answering why it's not worth knowing your skin type. The truth is that any attempt to categorize your skin as oily, dry, acne-prone, etc. is absolutely useless. The opposite is true—it creates even more problems (producers of cosmetics are more than happy to suggest a variety of products to fight those problems, too).

AFTER READING CHAPTER FIVE

you'll learn how to choose a suitable cream or serum. Choosing beauty products seems like a long and complicated task. The products suggesting unbelievable results for your skin are abundant. But if we look at the facts and scientific research, we'll see that only a few skin care product ingredients are truly effective (the rest of them, unfortunately, are just theories and suppositions). Knowing which ingredients to look for brings you a sense of relief. The good news is that only three ingredients will solve many problems and are guaranteed to improve your skin. However, some of them have side effects which you need to know about. We'll discuss all of that in this chapter.

IN CHAPTER SIX

we'll talk about the secrets of moisturizing your skin. It's one of the most important steps in skin care, so I decided to talk about this topic separately. Product supply is abundant, so naturally, it is difficult to choose. We'll discuss which six moisturizers are the best, and which ingredients should be avoided. I will also share my painful experience—how much money I wasted while looking for the perfect moisturizer.

CHAPTER SEVEN

is dedicated to helping you get rid of dull facial skin. Children's skin regenerates itself every three to four weeks. Dead skin cells shed and are replaced by new and vibrant ones. But as the time passes, the process slows down: the skin starts losing its glow and looks wrinkled because dead skin cells don't reflect the light.

That's why your face looks dull. In this chapter, we will talk in detail about the steps you could take or the products you could use to improve a natural skin regeneration process so that you can enjoy your beautiful and glowing complexion again!

CHAPTER EIGHT

is going to be one of the most important ones in this book! All I can say is that any step you take to preserve your youth and beauty will be ineffective if you ignore this important rule. A while ago, this topic did not interest me; however, everything changed when I met this beautiful girl while living in Los Angeles. Her skin was enviable despite the fact that she was older than me. It's been 20 years since the day she revealed the secret of her beauty and youthfulness. Based on my experience, I can confirm that she was right. Maybe it's time you apply this rule to your life?

IN CHAPTER NINE

we'll discuss how to solve skin care problems: how to get rid of acne, blackheads, dark spots, fine lines and wrinkles, dark circles under eyes, and how to get back your firm and glowing skin. We will also talk in detail about how you could become friends with your skin, whether it is oily, dry, or sensitive. Your skin care routine is very important when your complexion is problematic. Even if it doesn't bother you, and you think this chapter may not be important, I still invite you to read it carefully as we will talk about the essence of skin care. Without this basic knowledge, you cannot expect to enjoy your beautiful, radiant, and smooth skin!

CHAPTER TEN

is dedicated to the nutrition that helps to preserve and enhance your beauty. We'll talk about the habits I developed at 30 which helped me to maintain a slim and healthy body, as well as beautiful skin. A while ago, when I had so many problems with my skin, specialists all over the world claimed in unison that problematic skin, youthfulness, and beauty have nothing to do with what you eat. What a mistake it is to believe that! The truth is that you can easily guess what a woman eats by looking at her face. The beauty of your skin directly depends on your nutrition. You can't ignore that! However, I want to assure you that I am not suggesting any diets (I have tried tons of them). I'll share with you my five habits which helped me to achieve desirable results and, finally, balanced my weight for good.

CHAPTER ELEVEN

is going to be about an invisible side of beauty. I thought long and hard about whether this chapter was necessary. What made me decide to write it is that a woman can use the best skin care products, she can be aware of all the secrets of external beauty, but still…she can be unattractive. I knew many women who looked like they had just stepped off the cover of the fashion magazine. Unfortunately, I wanted to run away from them as soon as they opened their mouth. That's why in this chapter, we'll go over some qualities which make women unattractive to men and other women. I singled out three qualities which every woman should get rid of as soon as possible. You'll become beautiful inside and out. That's what I wish for you the most!

BUT ALSO,

in this book I will reveal skin care secrets and tried and true scientific facts. As cosmetic products are consistently being developed and perfected, I am not going to mention any specific names.

I have put all of the information into a separate PDF book, which will constantly be updated based on the latest product innovations and technologies.

You can order an electronic book in PDF format following the link below:

www.chocolate4soul.com/BookReport

CONTENTS

Chapter ONE

How we age ourselves prematurely without even knowing it

I thought long and hard about how to begin this book. I decided I wanted to start by sharing with you my most important message. During an interview on a TV show, I was asked about the main obstacle that stands in the way of Lithuanian women being beautiful, happy, and youthful.

At that time, my thoughts were all over the place. I wanted to say something intelligent. I thought to myself that maybe it was the lack of knowledge, motivation, or even money?

I was about to open my mouth and give some trivial answer when the right answer crossed my mind—we create obstacles by believing and talking about "ships that have sailed."

While talking to women from other countries, I often noticed that we Lithuanians tend to criticize ourselves more than we should. Unlike women of other nationalities, we seem eager to "write ourselves off" all too soon as no longer young and beautiful. So as strange as it may sound, the answer is that we get in our own way.

The time has come to re-evaluate our beliefs, the *gifts* we have inherited from our parents and society, that block us from preserving our beauty and youth. At the risk of sounding unpleasant, may I remind you that by being a part of a society, we adopt many of its beliefs and conventions. But we must understand that even though they occupy our minds, they are not *ours*. They are squatters that belong to our parents and the society we come from.

These thoughts and various *truths about life* were planted in our brains as children. We believed them then, and now we have made them our own. But they don't have to be.

THE STANDARD SET OF BELIEFS PASSED ON FROM ONE GENERATION TO THE NEXT

When I started my semi-independent life, my vision and expectations for my future were predictably already mapped out.

I had to find a husband as soon as possible since the idea of becoming an old maid was unbearable. I also believed that I wouldn't be young forever, so I had to act fast. Every birthday meant that my beauty was fading, and my health would soon start deteriorating too.

Becoming 40 was horrifying to me, as women of that age seemed old and boring. It was common in my environment to hear a popular warning about the *ship that had sailed*, so I couldn't miss it. To tell you the truth, for many years, I felt like I was becoming an old lady. I feared losing my beauty and health before even fully enjoying them. That annoying idea of the sailed ship drove me crazy and was always in the back of my mind.

My views have completely changed since then, but I had to put a lot of effort into changing them for that to happen. These beliefs are so deep-seated in our minds that, most of the time, we never question their truthfulness.

I constantly talk to women, and I can say without hesitation that not a day goes by without hearing a woman make a derisive comment about herself or a self-deprecating joke about her old age or something being *too late*. Since we are so accustomed to this, we don't even hear how often we repeat it and just keep reprogramming ourselves.

Not long ago, while talking to a friend, I was silently counting how many times she reminded herself that she had no more expectations since, at 30, she was already going downhill.

"You understand, Ruta, that at my age it's inappropriate to run marathons or have babies. I am not a spring chicken anymore, and I have to remember that. Nobody is getting younger."

The woman kept repeating it. However, she didn't stop there and went on to say, "If I didn't start it earlier, it's definitely not the time now. Not at my age. Who needs an old maid in her forties? Who?"

Her final statement was, "I am not technologically savvy, let's leave that to young people." These ideas ran through the entire conversation, and she seemed to be longing for the past. An hour later, the person facing me was not my beautiful friend, but a woman without any joy of living left in her, who was watching her *ship sail away*.

At first glance, these statements seem harmless, don't they? So what if you hint at life slipping through your fingers? But this is not innocent, because you are aging yourself prematurely and consistently convincing yourself that your time is up.

NEVER FORGET THAT OUR BODY HEARS WHAT OUR LIPS ARE SAYING

I am not about to open a discussion about the power of beliefs; suffice it to say that we are constantly programming ourselves, which is completely unnecessary.

I can without a doubt share with you one very important observation: while traveling around the world throughout my life, I noticed that women who express that point of view look much worse than those who believe that they can do anything and that their life is just beginning. I won the lottery because one of these positive women is my mother.

On my 20th birthday, as soon as I started talking about fine lines and how time flies, my mother quickly cut me off by saying that her beauty bloomed in her 30's. Later, it turned out that her beauty actually bloomed in her 40's. And on my 40th birthday, my mother claimed that, frankly, she felt her most beautiful and wonderful in her 50's!

When I look at my mother, I see that she is an incredibly beautiful and youthful woman. Her beauty is timeless. And that is true because my mother believes that the coming years will be even better and more interesting.

Later, when I left Lithuania, I met many women with sparkling eyes who enjoyed the gifts of life with a smile and much appreciation. I enjoyed prodding them to see how they thought and what fed their minds.

You'll probably guess that none of them mentioned *sailed ships* or complained about an aching back, a clear sign of a deteriorating body. Not even once did they mention that they were not getting younger!

I liked to tease my gorgeous friends since I was itching to know if they would buy into beliefs about aging or let them slide.

Once, I complained about my worrisome teeth with a sigh. "You know, since I turned 35, everything has started to fall apart. My teeth and joints . . . There is nothing you can do about aging," I blurted out to a friend.

I can still see her eyes wide open with surprise. She responded, "You're kidding me. My friend's 16-year-old daughter has more problems with dental fillings and joints than you do. What does age have to do with that, Ruta?"

Her words were a welcomed lesson for me. I realized that the smallest things do not have to be caused by aging.

Since then, I have searched and compiled many different answers. Now, while standing in front of the mirror looking for that wrinkled

40-year-old lady, I hear another inner voice telling me, "Some 20-year-olds have more fine lines than I do, so I just have to make sure that my skin is moisturized, check if my undereye concealer has ingredients drying my skin, get a good night's sleep, and go on with my life."

JOKES ABOUT YOUR AGE ARE AGING YOU AS WELL

I often notice women joking, "Oops, I can't remember such-and-such. Well, what can I do? With age, your memory gets worse." They say this without even thinking, quite unconsciously.

But we can think and speak completely differently. Children often forget things as well, but it never occurs to us to blame the *sailed ships they missed*. I wonder why we do this to ourselves. Why do we rob ourselves, bit by bit, day by day, of our own beauty and youth?

BUILDING AN INNER ORDER AND REPLACING OLD BELIEFS

1. Learn to recognize when and how you harm yourself

For a few days or weeks, watch yourself and others. Everything that stands in the way of your feeling young and beautiful will gradually begin to stand out and come fully into view.

By listening to your parents, friends, and people around you, you will quickly learn which sets of beliefs were passed on to you, and how you talk to yourself.

After I began observing myself more closely, I was horrified to discover that almost every other thought was self-criticism or doubt about my value and capabilities.

With time, I got to know my inner content so well that, just by looking at another woman, I could see what was on her mind. It's quite obvious.

If our lives don't resemble the ones we dreamt of, it means there is something inside of us preventing that from happening. There is no way around it: if you want to have a beautiful garden, you must begin by weeding it, and only then can you plant new seeds, right?

In other words, I suggest that you not repeat statements based on preconceived notions. And if you hear someone try to convince you of these "truths," intentionally let them go in one ear and out the other.

Sometimes, while sitting across from a person, I carefully listen to their choice of words. As soon as I hear the phrases *it's not going to happen, you shouldn't dress like that, you are a middle-aged woman, you should be OK with declining health,* or anything of the kind, I imagine a baseball bat in my hand pounding on those sneaky statements.

If any of them affect me more than expected, I start questioning if there is any truth to them. What's interesting is that I am convinced time and time again that there is no truth to them, only the views and interpretations of different people.

2. Convictions are neither truths nor lies. They are beliefs.

We should store in our minds only useful beliefs, while rejecting and neutralizing the rest as soon as possible.

I am presently 42 and expecting my second daughter. We have tried to conceive her for three years. I am sure she wouldn't be on the way if I had listened to all the doctors talking about my age, old eggs, and age-related dangers.

Remember—only after shedding old beliefs will you be able to fulfill your dreams. This shift frees women to create their own lives. The process happens more easily and faster than we imagine.

Later, we will discuss taking advantage of this new point of view and convincing ourselves that we are timeless. But for now, let's skip a few steps and look at how we get in our own way and lie to ourselves.

Beliefs often masquerade as useful and convenient. Let's say that we believe that women's metabolisms slow down with age, and that's why they gain weight. If we believe that, we stop trying and give up. It's a convenient statement, isn't it?

Women who feel lazy about taking care of their face would rather believe they lost in the genetic lottery than change their habits and finally get to know their skin. What's the point in taking care of your face if you believe the inevitable will happen?

What can we do when we are surrounded by so many obviously false beliefs?

Clearly, we meet people who age prematurely, have a variety of diseases at an early age, become obese, and so on.

But it's important to remember one basic fact: you vibrate at the same frequency that grabs your attention and energy. Remember that false beliefs will always exist and will be passed on from one generation to the next.

Only you can decide which ones are worthy of your attention and energy, and which ones should be acknowledged and dismissed. Our body will follow our thoughts and beliefs. There is no way around it. Taking care of your body is a life-long task. It's a waste of time to look for ways out of it, to label yourself as someone who is already aging or has bad genes.

3. New evidence that we were wrong

As soon as you decide to get rid of old beliefs, they start losing their grip on you. If you want to speed up changes, you must give your mind a helping hand by convincing it that it's OK to change direction. You have to give it permission to do so.

If you look around, you will see youthful, radiant women enjoying their life. When it was convenient not to notice them, when you were holding on to your old beliefs, you probably didn't see them. Now that you are ready, your inner changes will happen quickly.

So now it's time to gather evidence.

When I was dreaming about having a baby, I watched short films on YouTube about Hollywood stars who were blessed with motherhood at 40. When I looked for the confirmation that I could be attractive, strong, and energetic at 50, I read Jennifer Lopez's stories or browsed the internet for her pictures.

It's possible to find many stories and examples; it's up to us to decide where we direct our attention.

4. A practical task to help you fulfill your dreams more quickly

Let me get ahead of myself for a moment.

Reading this book, you will learn about the skin care problems I dealt with most of my life.

For the longest time, I was convinced that my skin would never be beautiful. My face had huge acne scars, my skin was dry and full of dreaded brown spots.

A psychologist suggested that I start reprogramming my mind by writing 50 times every morning: "My skin is smooth and beautiful." I experienced enormous resistance to the exercise. I did, however, overcome it and eventually started writing: "My skin is getting more beautiful and smooth every day."

I can't say this is the best kind of skin treatment, but this simple sentence gave me hope and helped counteract my daily habit of saying negative things about my skin when looking in the mirror.

The sentences I repeated daily motivated me to look for new ways to help my skin regain its glow and beauty.

With time, I fell in love with affirmations and understood their magic. That's why right now, when I want to convince myself of something, I take a pen and piece of paper in the morning, and I write down the words that give me strength 20 times in a row.

While I was pregnant, I wrote this sentence every morning: "There is a strong and healthy baby growing inside my body." I kept writing it until my anxiety disappeared.

Not long ago, I started my morning writings about having strong and healthy hair since I had unintentionally convinced myself that it was impossible. In the last few weeks, I noticed that the affirmation magic has started to work. I am choosing better product combinations, and I often take the time for scalp massages and other things that were blocked by my false beliefs.

5. Accept compliments and enjoy yourself

Here is one more useful piece of advice. Sometimes you naturally find yourself in what I would call a "beauty zone." I am referring to moments that occur accidentally or are created by others: a compliment from an important man or a stranger, or maybe just a flood of pleasant comments under your picture on a social network.

Enjoy those moments when you become beautiful and youthful again, and the future seems wonderful and bright. Indulge in them as long as you can. We all need help and support to see ourselves as gorgeous and wonderful women. Allow yourself to feel joy, as opposed to denying your beauty or downplaying a compliment or sincere comment.

Beginning in childhood, many of us women internalized the idea that we must put ourselves down and criticize ourselves. That's why, when we are on our way to a brighter future, we have to learn to treat ourselves differently. The more we enjoy our achievements, the sooner we see the desired results.

In this chapter, we talked about beauty; however, I suggest that you apply this valuable information to other areas of your life as well. If, after taking a closer look at your life, you notice that some areas don't bring you joy, don't be afraid to take a closer look at yourself. You are very likely to find many stumbling blocks in your thoughts and actions that don't allow you to enjoy and fulfill your dreams.

Every woman can explore herself and change her beliefs. The fact that you got this book and have just read this chapter shows your determination and readiness. Don't stop!

Chapter **TWO**

Constant disappointments with skin problems,
and great discoveries that changed everything

In the previous chapter, we discussed beliefs and learned that to get good results, we have to change our attitude and rid ourselves of inner limitations.

Our thoughts greatly affect us, but their power is not enough to make us become young and beautiful. On their own, self-talk and our inner voice won't make us achieve the goal of becoming happy and satisfied. We need knowledge. To be more specific, we need the right information. Besides, we must understand the basic principles of body and skin care so that we can find the right products in the vast ocean of excessive supply. It was probably difficult to find quality facial creams, shampoos, or body washes 50 years ago. But today, the situation is the opposite; the supply is so plentiful that you can waste a lifetime spending money on ineffective products without ever achieving the desired results. That's the best-case scenario. The worst-case scenario is that you might create more problems by damaging your skin.

My journey to achieving beautiful, glowing skin was long and arduous. It goes back to a time when people in my country knew very little about skin care problems and their solutions.

THE PAIN OF ACNE

As soon as I reached the age of 14, my face broke out in zits, and blackheads appeared on my nose and chin. My mother brought me to a cosmetologist who took on the hard job of rescuing my skin.

Even now I can remember facial steamers, cheese cloth, the painful popping of zits and blackheads, and the constant smell of rubbing alcohol. It was followed by a drying mask with camphor intended to "disinfect and minimize my pores." After this painful treatment, I used to drag myself home in tears.

And then the "healing" was supposed to start. I hid myself indoors because I was ashamed to show my face. After the procedures with the rubbing alcohol and other drying ingredients, my face became even more oily, so much so that every time I looked in the mirror, I cried even more.

Unfortunately, a week later, my acne would become infected again, and my mother would take me back to the cosmetologist. My heart breaks when I think of those times. Oh, how I wish someone would have explained to me that this type of skin "care" would leave scars on my face and in my heart.

Anyone who has had severe acne will understand me: I wanted to cry every time I looked at my skin. My self-confidence was non-existent, and dates with boys were extremely uncomfortable as the only thought on my mind was, "Is he disgusted by me or not?"

I would talk with my head turned away, and under no circumstances would I allow someone to touch my skin.

DISAPPOINTING EFFORTS TO
GET RID OF MY SKIN PROBLEMS

With each passing year, my skin condition worsened. The little scars multiplied, and my skin was not only oily but also wrinkly. I frequented tanning salons to try to cover my utter shame. Unfortunately, long-term tanning did not do me any good either—I just got more fine lines and blemishes, and my skin looked tired. Sometimes I experienced painful, infected zits which required drainage. I would do nothing but cry for days on end.

That's what I endured until I was about 28.

During that period, I traveled around the world a few times, meeting many cosmetologists and dermatologists and spending a lot of money on their treatments and products.

Every specialist gave me fresh hope and faith that this was definitely going to help me. Unfortunately, the results were always short-lived. In no time at all, I would find myself looking for a better product, a better specialist, and a more effective magic pill.

At that time, I was traveling around the world and making good money. At first, I worked as a model—I was lucky because photographers noticed my unique facial features and ignored my problem skin.

At 14, I started working as a photo model for a highly respected and beloved photographer. His photographs were published in popular Lithuanian magazines.

Later, I had modelling jobs in other European countries, but to tell you the truth, they never brought me joy. I received interesting and lucrative offers but, unfortunately, I didn't feel beautiful and confident.

I got tired of the job and became a waitress on cruise ships traveling around the world. That's how I made my living and saved enough money for my condo and, of course, my never-ending facial care products.

I must admit that when I started traveling and working, I stopped buying creams and visiting cosmetologists—I just lost faith in their usefulness. I started spending money on different foundation creams and concealers and learned to mask my acne under a thick layer of powder.

At that time, I had no idea about a healthy lifestyle. My emotions and disappointments were drowned in red wine and cigarettes, and I just couldn't be bothered anymore.

As it happens, in my travels, I was given advice by women from different countries. I tried a variety of acne-fighting remedies and occasionally trusted some special facial care product line, containing some magic Brazilian berries or a miraculous nut oil sold by a rough-handed woman from Papua New Guinea. Oh, I could also mention the herbs over which an old Chinese lady cast a spell. They irritated my skin a few times. I think you get the picture.

As sad as it is to admit, I looked much worse at 22 than I do today at 42. My tired, dull, acne-covered, and blemished skin was really a problem, and it was poisoning my life.

When I look through my old pictures, I see a tired young woman with no radiance in her eyes.

CHANGES FROM THE CITY OF ANGELS

A modeling agency invited me to work in Los Angeles, so I packed my bags and left for the City of Angels. At first it was difficult. All the money I earned went to the lawyers dealing with my immigration status so I could work legally, pay my taxes, and have a place under the Californian sun.

Unfortunately, they failed to convince the US Embassy how unique and useful I was for this country, and the only way to remain in the United States was to get married. So I conveniently got married. I am not proud of my fake marriage, but I must admit that it quickly changed my life for the better.

Suddenly, I had more money and time to invest in skin care and learning. However, when it came to applying this new information, I took my time because what I wanted more than anything else was to find the *silver bullet* that would get rid of all my skin problems.

For the next few years, I spent money on different products, pills, teas, and supplements.

I visited the best dermatologists in Beverly Hills, and they all repeated the same thing: food has nothing to do with your problem, you just have to choose appropriate products. I trusted the *miracle workers* and waited for the miracle.

Unfortunately, more money and better doctors did not solve my problems. My bathroom cabinet was filled to the brim with expensive facial products, but my face was still covered in acne. My skin was dull and blemished.

When someone tells me that I am lucky to have such beautiful skin, I want to laugh and cry at the same time. The situation only improved when I finally took responsibility for my appearance and self-esteem and started looking for science-based facts.

I probably know more than most women and girls do about what it means to put yourself down and pull yourself back up again. I have done it so many times.

EXTREME ACTIONS TO IMPROVE MY SKIN

My last attempt, in a long series of attempts to improve my skin, focused on taking a strong medication used for the treatment of acne. (That particular medication known as Accutane was later banned in the United States because of harmful side effects.) My doctor in Los Angeles declined to prescribe this medication because I smoked, used contraceptive pills, had anemia, and experienced constant anxiety and mood swings.

But I would not be deterred. I travelled to Mexico to buy the miracle medication. I was utterly convinced it would heal my skin. By then, I was truly desperate and ready to do anything to have beautiful skin.

After taking the medication for about six months, not only did my complexion undergo serious changes, but so did my mental health: my skin became red and sensitive to the sun, and my mood swings increased, but I kept going, hoping that this medication would get rid of the acne which had bothered me for so many years.

I am not going to lie—the medication did help. But what upsets me is the fact that what I know now would have helped me deal with my skin problems in a much simpler, easier, and faster way.

So, what happened? The horrible acne finally disappeared, but it left many scars, wrinkles, and blemishes on my skin. My skin lost any youthful firmness it had managed to preserve, and I did not know what to do next.

That's when I became really angry. I decided to forget about any advice I heard and give up on cosmetologists, who could barely help me anyway. I decided to enroll in a beauty school in Glendale.

LESSONS FROM BEAUTY SCHOOL

I ended up enrolling in a beauty school in Los Angeles and, at first, I found the lessons really frustrating since the main instructor, a lady from Thailand, loved to talk about meditation, food, and other annoying subjects. She drove me crazy for the first few months!

I paid big bucks and I wanted to learn how to become more beautiful, not stare at a rose bud while sitting by the ocean or enjoy a quick cell regeneration by walking outdoors.

Eventually I gave in, and my attitude started to change completely. For the first time, my mind got a fresh perspective and I saw my body as a whole.

The next year, I did extensive research about skin, became a licensed beautician, and worked in different clinics in Los Angeles, all the while collecting valuable knowledge. I invested a lot of time and money into this: I attended the best seminars, analyzed product contents during my evenings, and kept working tirelessly.

New knowledge gave me mixed feelings. On some days, I felt really angry because I had been fooled for so many years. Sometimes I felt sad for the wasted time and money. At other times, I was looking for someone to blame for this mess.

I spent a year testing various treatments, procedures and products on myself, my colleagues, and my clients. Finally, I figured out what really worked, and what was just a manufacturer's gimmick. I was quite surprised to learn that there are very few products that are actually effective.

Beauty school was valuable to me. Sometimes I jokingly say that I was very lucky to have the chance to study in two different worlds. The Asian attitude towards skincare focuses mostly on prevention, while Americans focus on innovations, facts, scientific research, and things of that nature.

In the morning lectures, the instructor would cover different preventative massage techniques she learned at the age of 10, while during the afternoon lectures, we listened to representatives of various cosmetic companies tell us about the newest cosmetic products and suggest free injections. Their goal was to prepare a new generation of cosmetologists to work with their products.

In time, I understood the effects of nutrition and movement on our beauty and our sense of well-being, so I decided to enter the National Academy of Sports Medicine. I'll discuss nutrition in more detail in a later chapter.

My skin was finally healing and clearing. Brown and red acne blemishes started to disappear. I avoided the sun and stopped tanning. My knowledge finally allowed me to choose appropriate and effective products. Even though the healing process was not as fast as I expected —I made many mistakes, learned from them, fine-tuned my approach and was often disappointed yet again—it was obvious to anyone that my skin condition was noticeably improving.

MY WISH FOR YOU IS GOOD RESULTS, FAST

I sincerely hope that with the advice you find in this book, you will improve your skin condition much faster than I did. If you apply my knowledge, you will notice the first results sooner than you might expect. But be patient—you will be proud of your well-cared-for skin in about six months. Today I am 42, and my skin condition is the best it has ever been. It's completely clear, healthy, and radiant. The little scars on my face are almost invisible. Of course, if you look really closely, you will detect spots where the acne used to be, but they are not enough to bother me.

I continue the intensive care of my skin because if I let it go and forget my own advice, its condition immediately worsens, and the pimples resurface sooner rather than later. But I am no longer afraid of my skin condition, as it motivates me to focus, re-examine my nutrition and the cosmetics I use, and invest time and effort into skin care.

After reading this book you will know how to deal with all these problems because I will share the discoveries I made that can lead to the ultimate goal of healthy skin in the shortest possible time.

You will also have all the knowledge you need to look more beautiful than today. Most importantly, you will learn to understand your skin and give it what it is asking for. That is the best and the most effective way to preserve beauty and youth.

Until you learn the basic truths, it will be very easy to fool you, talk you into buying useless products, and make you dependent on the false advice and services of many cosmetologists.

The next chapter is the continuation of my story, a journey full of twists and turns. We'll discuss beauty myths and the plain lies that made me waste a lot of time and money. Before I started to write the next chapter, I planned to mention no more than 10 points. But after having written 27 of them, I realized that I still had not reached the end! It made me really sad to see how long I was fooled. My consolation is that your road could be much shorter and easier.

Chapter THREE

The cosmetics industry myths and little white lies
that made me waste tons of money and time

This chapter may be a little technical, but it is highly informative and necessary. If we want to understand which "inventions" of the beauty industry are effective, we must spend some time learning what is ineffective. Only after we analyze mistakes can we critically evaluate our choices in the future.

It's very important to talk openly about beauty myths because I see so many women around me making the same mistakes I did. Besides, we live in a time of booming social networks, and they do a good job convincing us to try new products that are questionable and often devoid of scientific evidence.

To understand the basics about our skin, we have to discuss the main myths, mistakes, and little white lies that are so widespread in the beauty and skin care industry.

1. THE MYTH ABOUT EYE CREAMS

Let's start with eye creams. There is a reason why the number of companies making eye creams is decreasing. They don't work.

There are no scientific studies or evidence proving that the eye area needs different ingredients than your face, neck, or cleavage. I wasted quite a lot of money on them just to learn that they are absolutely useless.

Any cream or serum containing plenty of antioxidants (we'll talk about them later), moisturizers, or vitamins is good for the eye area. We don't have to pay double for a separate container labelled eye cream.

If I feel that my undereye area is getting dry, I focus on it. I apply some good serum with hyaluronic acid and antioxidants, and seal in the moisture and other important ingredients with a simple fragrance-free moisturizing cream. We'll go over the whole skin care routine in the following chapters, so I will not go into too much detail here.

2. THE MYTH ABOUT SWITCHING PRODUCTS OFTEN

In the past and for the longest time, I used to regularly switch products because I was convinced that my skin got used to them and they lost their efficacy. Now, after discovering reliable quality products, I have been using the same ones for several years. Of course, I remain interested in learning about the most recent innovations in the field of cosmetics and skin care, but this doesn't mean I throw out the baby with the bathwater.

If I discover a more effective product, I say goodbye to the old one, not because a friend or an influencer suggested it, but because its effectiveness has been scientifically proven.

I don't do it because my skin gets used to it. That's a myth. It's been proven that our skin renews itself every 30 days, so brand-new skin cells interact with the product for the first time.

Our skin most certainly does not get used to these products. If we followed this logic, the benefits of eating vegetables would reach a plateau after a while. But we know that eating fruits and vegetables is always healthy and that our body does not get used to them, so why should it get used to a serum or a cream?

Skin is no different than any other organ. Of course, it could be beneficial to go back and forth between serums since they have different vitamins and antioxidants. Also, as seasons change, I adjust my skin care routine to adapt to the cooler or warmer weather. But the same moisturizing creams and sunscreen products can be used for a long time.

3. THE MYTH ABOUT WASHING YOUR FACE OFTEN

I used to cleanse my oily skin two or three times a day. I liked products with a good lather, which left my skin feeling fresh. I believed that cleansing it often helped me avoid oiliness and made my pores look smaller. Unfortunately, the facts are different. The more we dry out our skin, the oilier it gets.

And the more oil there is in the pores, the higher the chance that the dirt, which gets into the pores, will stick to their walls, mix with dead cells and oil, and cause new infections.

Now I clean my skin with a gentle moisturizing wash. And I also use microfiber washcloths.

If anyone asked me what helped me the most on my road to a more beautiful and healthier skin, I would answer in a heartbeat: appropriate cleansing and sunscreen, which we'll talk about in detail in the following chapters.

4. THE LIE ABOUT ACIDS

I used to be afraid of acids, as I was sure that using them would harm me. I thought acids were meant only for cosmetic clinics. However, that's not true. After I learned to use acids and "became friends" with them, I achieved really good results.

Appropriately selected acid exfoliates dead skin cells, induces skin regeneration, and erases facial blemishes and fine lines faster than any other product.

After reading this book, you will know exactly how to choose and use at least a few types of acids. They will help you achieve a genuine and obvious change in your complexion.

5. THE MYTH ABOUT EXPENSIVE COSMETICS

I dare not think about how much money I spent on expensive and completely useless cosmetics. Like many, if not most, women, I was convinced that expensive skin care products had a higher quality and worked better.

The fact is, there are only a few ingredients that are truly effective, research-based, and time-tested, and the beauty industry knows them all. All the other "magical" additives are just for merchandising, clever presentations, fragrances, and other unimportant tricks completely unrelated to the product efficacy.

Research studies have found and confirmed many times that a cream costing $10 can be much more effective than a serum costing $200.

After learning to read product ingredients, I was surprised. Expensive creams I paid hundreds of dollars for were full of skin irritating ingredients: essential oils, eucalyptus, and peppermint fragrances, for example. In the creams, I saw a lot of unnecessary paraffin and other substances whose only purpose is to extend the shelf life of the product.

I am not going to argue—they are very pleasant to use, and they smell fantastic. However, our skin is an organ, so our main concern should be a product's chemical formula, not presentation or packaging. That's why

I am not surprised that, after so many years of using expensive products, I still did not achieve optimal results.

I did, however, rid myself of the idea that I was missing out by applying a $10 cream or serum on my skin.

6. THE MYTH ABOUT MAKEUP WIPES AND MICELLAR WATER

For many years, I cleansed my face with different types of makeup wipes and micellar water because I was convinced that a better way to remove makeup simply did not exist. I don't like to think about how I would rub my face with a strange mix of preservatives and fragrances, believing that I was helping my skin.

Now I can say with certainty that the only thing worse than using makeup wipes is going to bed without removing your makeup at all.

Micellar water is a slightly better choice than not cleansing your face at all, but it's far from being a substitution for cleansing your face carefully with appropriately chosen cleansers and water (we'll learn how to choose them in later chapters). After a closer analysis of micellar water, I realized that when you use it to clean your face, the effect is like putting your hands in soapy water and then drying them off. I would only use micellar water while traveling with no opportunity to take a shower.

I don't use makeup wipes anymore since they don't remove dirt, and constant rubbing irritates the skin and spreads infections. The contents of the wipes are unhealthy, as they leave a film on your face that prevents your skin from breathing.

7. THE MYTH ABOUT NATURAL PRODUCTS

Another mistake I made was following the natural products fad and absolutely ignoring the chemistry behind all cosmetic and skin care products. At one point, I believed that if I didn't use any chemical ingredients, my skin would be even more beautiful.

Now I can unreservedly say that all the discussions about the benefits of natural ingredients are ill-founded. They are just another money-driven media hype.

If you knew the requirements allowing manufacturers to write the word "natural" on their packaging, you would be really disappointed. You would see that there are many ways to manipulate this requirement without telling the whole truth. It's almost impossible to know which part of the cream is made from natural components, and which one is created by scientists in laboratories.

They can argue that their cream consists of oils or butters for the most part. But how would they respond to my question: how was it created? After a lengthy discussion, we would probably end up going around in circles and the very possibility of the existence of a natural product would come into question. But more interestingly still, the question that is raised is: can it be good? Maybe it's so natural that it can breed bacteria that will do more harm than good.

Another thing that you may not want to hear is that there is no actual evidence that a natural or organic product brings better results. Often the opposite is true. Many irritating ingredients can be found in so-called natural skin care products.

Here is my current attitude toward *naturalness*: I am learning to read labels and appreciate technological innovations. I truly like wonderful and effective synthetic elements like hyaluronic acid, collagen, ceramides, glycerides, amino acids, retinols, and so on. There are many more synthetic ingredients, but I don't like them because I am not sure about the benefits they provide. That's why I try to make sure they are not on the labels of the products I use.

I also appreciate different oils and plant-based butters that I use almost every day. They soften my skin, supply it with antioxidants, and protect it against environmental factors. Unfortunately, natural products sometimes contain essential oils and other unwanted, irritating substances, so we shouldn't blindly trust the label "natural." Natural does not mean devoid of all sorts of chemicals; it just means perhaps a different sort of chemical.

Here is my advice: let's all learn to read labels, observe our skin, and see what it needs. Instead of going to extremes, let's use the best of both worlds, synthetic and natural. That's exactly what we are going to learn to do in this book.

8. THE MYTH ABOUT UNLIMITED WATER DRINKING

For several years, I drank water non-stop to moisturize my skin from the inside. I made myself drink at least 3 liters a day.

Unfortunately, the miracle didn't happen—I constantly ran to the bathroom, washed the minerals out of my body, and kept spending money on bottled water.

After seeking out the benefits of water, I finally realized that a greater amount of it would not make my skin more beautiful. By all means, I don't want to discourage you from drinking it. I just want to warn you that everything is good in moderation and should be in response to the needs of your body. It doesn't matter if your skin is dry or oily, it won't become hydrated just because you drink more water.

I finally came to this conclusion: the most important thing is balance. Extremes do us no favors. The best we can do for our skin is listen to it, learn to meet its needs, and develop healthy habits. After that, we will be on the right path, and soon everything will fall into place.

9. THE MYTH ABOUT NIGHT CREAMS

For the longest time, any moisturizing cream that I applied in the evening absolutely had to be labelled "night cream." It was the same mistake I made with eye creams and cleavage creams!

What should be the difference between a day and a night cream? It may simply be that a day cream should include an SPF. That's all.

I now have selected a few really good moisturizers to provide and preserve moisture in my skin. I apply the same basic cream in the daytime and at night. If I see that my skin needs more nourishment, I apply a few layers. If I need just a little bit of moisturizing, I apply a thin layer on a wet face. That helps me lock in the moisture without additional oil. In my morning routine, I never forget one important thing—sunscreen. That is probably one of the most important secrets of beautiful skin. I'll give you more details in later chapters.

10. THE MYTH OF BECOMING LIKE OUR PARENTS

For many years I believed that, by looking at our parents, we could imagine what we would look like at their age. Only much later did I finally understand that that is simply not the case. Of course, we inherit genes from them, but there are many more important factors that determine our skin condition and body shape.

Let's say, for example, that your mother didn't use sunscreen and loved sunbathing, while you never left the house without applying a sunscreen first. Chances are your skin will look much better than your mother's at the same age.

The same is true of the shape of our body down the road. We often copy our parents' eating habits and lifestyle, so our appearance is often caused, not by genes, but by habits. If your eating and exercise habits are healthier than your parents', it's very likely that your body will be in better shape than theirs too.

It doesn't make sense to convince yourself that you will have the same problems as your parents did, or to blame fate or genes for outcomes in your life that depend on actions you have taken over your lifetime.

11. THE MYTH ABOUT OILY SKIN AND MOISTURIZERS

For several years, I didn't use moisturizers or serums because I decided that oily skin didn't need moisturizing. After looking into scientific studies, I realized I was wrong.

Oily skin produces more oil than dry skin, but it still needs moisture. If you have dry skin and use moisturizers, especially if they are oil-free or silicone-based, your skin will look better in just two weeks.

Well-moisturized oily skin becomes balanced and stops making excessive amounts of oil. The pores finally become cleaner, literally shrink, and the number of pimples and blackheads dramatically decreases.

12. THE MYTH ABOUT POPULAR SUPPLEMENTS

I still can't quite understand why I wasted so much money on vitamin supplements.

For many years, I even drank collagen, which was nothing but a waste of money. After I studied the scientific literature, research results, and facts, I learned that drinkable collagen has barely any value at all. The same is true of most supplements.

Research shows that, after drinking collagen for a few weeks, a slight increase of collagen in your skin will be barely noticeable, if at all, and it will disappear as soon as you stop taking it.

It's not worth jumping on the bandwagon of taking supplements and similar products—probiotics, collagen, hyaluronic supplements, and skin enhancing teas. The effectiveness of these products has not been scientifically proven, and they are just one more waste of money.

The most important thing is a balanced diet full of vitamins, antioxidants, protein, and healthy fats. Our bodies will make all the other necessary elements.

I endorse what I consider to be reliable manufacturers whose philosophy I agree with: Solgar, Ritual, and Garden of Life whose representatives promote a wholesome attitude towards health and the world in general. The contents of their products are trustworthy, and most importantly, they don't include ingredients our bodies don't need.

Every two months, I buy vitamins for my family and myself. I try to base my choice on blood tests and understanding what our bodies really need. Usually these are iron supplements, vitamin D, different vitamin combinations, and so on. Sometimes, if we experience digestive or bowel movement problems, I buy reliable probiotics. I never spend money on fashionable or faddish products such as supplements recommended by influencers or celebrities, which are probably just advertisements in disguise, especially when the product is packed with sweeteners, preservatives, and other useless mixtures.

Occasionally, I see young women in social media getting shots of collagen, and it really upsets me. I know that these products are useless. I just hope that they aren't harmful as well.

But let's be clear. This is not a local problem. It's a worldwide problem. Did you know that many products that are classified as supplements in some countries have not been the subject of serious research and their effectiveness has not been scientifically proven? If manufacturers want to sell medications, they must include on their package label not just the list of benefits of the product, but the real and potentially harmful side effects as well.

It's a different story with supplements and cosmetics. There are no strict requirements. Manufacturers mention harmless ingredients and create their own impressive descriptions. The phrase "research-based" means that a small group of people tried the product. The tests are paid for by manufacturers themselves, so you can't expect an objective opinion.

I am so angry at myself for having stuffed my body with suspicious "new generation collagens" and other similar substances for so many years, thus making my liver constantly overwork and filter useless chemicals. I did it without examining the facts first. To make matters worse, after buying into the benefits of some products, I convinced my mother and my friends to use them as well. It's a shame, but I can't turn back the clock.

The best we can all do right now is not jump hastily in line to use trendy products, but take the time to examine them. These days, we can always Google a product and, after examining reviews, come to a decision based on rational thoughts and information, not just emotions.

13. THE MYTH ABOUT TONERS

Another big mistake I made was wasting money on toners. They seemed so necessary. Many years ago, cosmetologists assured me that when we cleanse our skin, the balance of acidity and alkalinity, what is called the pH balance, changes and a toner is necessary to restore that balance. At that time, I didn't have enough knowledge to discuss the topic of skin acidity, so I dutifully used a toner and tried to convince myself of its usefulness.

However, science says that toners are an unnecessary product: the skin care industry has improved considerably, and cleansers are not strong enough or aggressive enough to disrupt the pH balance or leave a film on the skin. Toners, in my view, are watery products with a few active ingredients and an unclear purpose. Unfortunately, most of them are worthless (and often harmful) to our skin. Toners usually include various fragrances, camphor, menthol, and other useless ingredients that dry out and irritate our skin.

Store shelves are overflowing with toner variations of all kinds: rose water, moisturizing essences, hyaluronic sprays, and so on.

If they don't contain skin irritating ingredients, there is no harm in using them. But it's important to remember that it's best to lock in moisture with an oil-free moisturizer or cream (we'll discuss this later).

On a hot summer day, ladies often use refreshing sprays without even thinking that water-based products wet your skin just for a short time. It quickly evaporates together with the moisture from your skin. So we need to decide for ourselves if we need toners or not. These days there are a lot of excellent serums and creams that help take care of our skin and preserve our youth. Think twice about whether you really need one watery product with a few active ingredients.

14. THE MYTH ABOUT HOMEMADE MASKS

I can't believe that I used to love homemade masks and made them almost every day. There was a time when I sincerely believed that by mixing aloe with honey and an egg, I could create a much more effective mask than the one I could find on a store shelf.

In all fairness, I must admit that the results were not so bad. The egg white would tighten my pores, the honey and aloe would moisturize my skin a little, and the effect was relatively obvious. But the only tangible results were temporarily softened skin.

At the beginning of this book, I openly shared with you the agony I went through with my skin. I was constantly searching for products that could help me and wouldn't make the situation worse.

Unfortunately, products from my fridge didn't improve my skin, and the problems didn't get solved. I finally started looking for scientific evidence and facts. When I couldn't find them, I learned that the content of homemade masks is often unclear, and food product molecules are often too big to penetrate the deeper skin layers and produce the desired effect. Our skin doesn't have the enzymes and acids necessary to process lemon or broccoli and transform them into beneficial vitamins to be absorbed rather than digested.

Homemade masks can also breed bacteria, as those mixtures don't have preservatives. If your skin is sensitive, bacteria is very likely to cause unwanted effects. Upon deeper analysis, it becomes clear that food products are meant for your stomach, not your skin.

Lately, I've been admiring scientific progress. Science allowed me to finally achieve the results I wanted. I appreciate the fact that scientists can take a lemon and aloe, extract their most beneficial components, and break them down to the smallest particles which can deeply penetrate the skin.

So, don't get me wrong: I don't mean to completely reject all products that you may find in your fridge. Aloe, avocado, or an egg can be somewhat beneficial. I just think that we'd be better off if we trust a reliable beauty product manufacturing company.

FOOD ITEMS TO AVOID PUTTING ON YOUR SKIN

Here is a list of some food products that you should never apply to your skin. I won't lie to you, I tried most of them, and I truly regret it.

Lemon. Like I said before, I used to love homemade masks and sometimes, thinking I was being smart, I would apply lemon juice to my face instead of buying vitamin C serum. As I felt my face tingling, I waited expectantly for a brightening, blemish-removing effect. My behavior was really foolish. I would never do that again. Lemon irritates your skin and changes its pH to acidic. Skin becomes sensitive to the sun, and the desired result is never obtained. It's better to find a reliable manufacturer and trust the vitamin C formula mixed in the lab.

Baking soda. Exfoliating cream made of baking soda was one of my favorites. I believed that it would help get rid of dead skin cells and give my skin a second life. The effect of baking soda is the opposite of lemon. Baking soda makes the pH of the skin more alkaline. After such treatments, irritated and stressed skin must work hard to restore its pH and create a new protective barrier.

Facial disinfection with rubbing alcohol. Yes, I considered rubbing alcohol my friend. I liked to disinfect my face with it and destroy acne bacteria. I used to pop facial zits and blackheads daily, followed by a serious disinfection with rubbing alcohol, vodka, cologne, or a similar liquid, and calmly walked into the backyard to dry off and heal my pimples in the sun. Everything seemed logical to me. Destroying bacteria with alcohol seemed effective, and the sun, so I thought at the time, was a gift of nature to speed up the healing process.

This lethal combination left me with brown spots so big and bright, it was impossible to hide them under the thickest layer of makeup. It hurts even to write about it! I have to apologize to my skin over and over again for practices like this.

Now I stay away from all alcohol-based products. Even when I wear perfume, I try not to spray my neck or cleavage area as I am afraid to see what I saw on my skin before.

Toothpaste. Unfortunately, this was one of my favorite products to treat my acne. Sometimes I would even make a little mask for especially pimply areas on my face.

Yes, I know, it doesn't sound very good. But I can swear that, at that time, these treatments seemed truly powerful. A pleasant cooling sensation of menthol signaled my brain that my skin was responding. I would start feeling a sense of cleanliness, a pleasant tingling, and was imagining how the toothpaste was removing all the pus in my zits.

Well, my love of toothpaste did not really make the situation worse, but the benefits were more imagined than real. Until one day when I put toothpaste on a very big pimple. The toothpaste ingredients irritated it so much that it grew into a large cyst that had to be drained two weeks later. The treatment left a huge scar on my face and a deep pain in my heart. I stayed at home for the longest time and went outside only with a large Band-Aid on my face.

So please, do not put toothpaste on your face. It has fluoride, menthol, and other substances for which your skin will never thank you. If you want to apply something to your pimple, let it be a product with BHA (salicylic acid), sulphur, or benzoyl peroxide, which we'll discuss later.

15. THE MYTH ABOUT SOAPS AND FEMININE WASHES

Soap. I used to wash my face with soap quite often. It seemed to me that it was the only product that could cleanse my face properly. This type of cleansing had a bad effect on my skin, but I ignored all the signals because I really liked the short-term effect of soap.

In actuality, soap dries out and irritates your skin. As the dried-out skin tries to regain its natural condition as soon as possible, it starts producing more oil. The oil clogs the pores. They start to gather more dirt, and more pimples appear. It's also worth mentioning that soap leaves the face covered with a film, which does not make your skin more beautiful and radiant. The ingredients that make the soap foam and keep its shape are definitely not beneficial to your skin.

Intimate areas. For many years, I washed my intimate areas with a variety of scented washes or antibacterial soaps. Much later I learned that I was making a huge mistake.

My intimate areas would constantly cause me problems. I couldn't get rid of recurring yeast and other unpleasant infections. I was a repeat customer in pharmacies and gynecological clinics, often visiting their offices and looking for an effective wash, vaginal tablet, or some kind of pill to take care of my problem. After a few years, I got tired of the ritual and started looking for ways to help myself.

My discoveries shocked me. It turns out that, thanks to my naivete and lack of knowledge, I was just caught in a vicious cycle.

I used perfumed products that were packed with sulfites and drying, irritating ingredients, hoping to feel clean and germ-free. Nonsense. It's no surprise that I became a frequent pharmacy customer. I just kept making the situation worse and worse, and there was no way out.

Not long ago, I was looking for a new feminine wash and went to a drugstore for suggestions. The two products specifically recommended to me by a pharmacist used SLS (sodium lauryl sulfate) as a base, an aggressive, drying vaginal foaming agent that destroys everything in its path, good and bad, and should have no place in feminine washes.

So if you want your intimates to be healthy, it's better to use a mild wash that has no SLS or fragrances. Make sure the product pH is 4.5 to 5.5, as the average of your intimate area should be more acidic to prevent bacteria from growing and proliferating.

I destroyed my pH with the alkaline wash. Bacteria immediately started to grow, and the next thing I knew, I was standing in line once again for vaginal tablets that only temporarily solved the problem. Then I started the cycle all over again in a few days thanks to the same washes. Not a good healing strategy. I don't want this for you.

16. THE MYTH ABOUT PILLOWS AND SLEEP

If I knew then what I know now, and could turn back the clock, I would have thrown away all the pillowcases made of cotton, flannel, polyester, you name it, a long time ago. In my early youth, I would have used pillowcases made out of a quality silk.

In the past, I would get a lot of acne when I used cotton. Your pillowcase becomes an incredible breeding ground for bacteria when your face sweats in your sleep. The situation improved when I started changing pillowcases every few days.

But now I rest my head strictly on silk pillowcases that I change only once a week because they don't allow bacteria to grow. Silk seems to have antibacterial properties.

I don't claim that all your acne and other skin problems will disappear when you sleep on silk, but I can guarantee that your skin and your hair will certainly look better. And here is why: silk absorbs much less moisture than cotton, so sleeping on it makes your skin look fresher and more radiant. Silk is also slower to absorb serums and creams, so the products you applied at night should remain on your face rather than transfer to your pillowcase.

I remember being really surprised to find that I did not have the usual pillow marks on my face after I started sleeping on silk. I so wish I would have known earlier what a difference it makes to sleep on silk. We spend about eight hours a night on a pillow. I think it's worth investing into high quality silk pillowcases.

For many years, my hair was no less problematic than my skin. It was weak, thinning, and prone to breakage. Sleeping on silk improved its appearance. Not only did it grow longer, but it was also smoother and stronger.

Now that I know the benefits of silk, I take my pillowcases with me when I go on a trip and slip them on as soon as I get to the hotel.

17. THE MYTH ABOUT NUTRITION AND YOUR SKIN

One of the biggest mistakes I made had to do with the belief that acne and other skin reactions had nothing to do with the food I ate.

The more time goes by, the less tolerant I become, and I have no respect for any cosmetologist, dermatologist, dentist, physician, or specialist in any related field who claims that food is not important for the condition of our skin or our overall health. I view these claims as warnings: no need to continue seeing these specialists since their opinions are not trustworthy.

I studied a detailed analysis of the effect of food on our hormone system, and how important it is for our skin and general well-being. Just by looking at a young woman's face, I now can guess what she eats.

Later we'll discuss in more detail how to determine which products you should limit to improve your skin.

Absolutely everything is related to our food and lifestyle: our emotions, mood, skin condition, sex drive, weight, and many other things.

There is more in a separate chapter about nutrition, so keep reading.

18. THE MYTH ABOUT CREAMS TO REDUCE FINE LINES

For many years I have been searching for a cream that would reduce wrinkles and fine lines, but I still haven't found one.

The truth is that no cream will ever eliminate your wrinkles. The structure of a wrinkle is such that no external cream will bring it back to its initial appearance. It's not worth buying expensive creams and hoping for a miracle.

I do have some good news, though. Wrinkles look deeper when the skin is dry and has an accumulation of dead skin cells, which don't reflect light. The same is true when skin lacks elasticity and firmness. Creams, serums, and acid masks chosen with discernment may help you fight those problems and make wrinkles look smaller. They may not necessarily be expensive, either.

My skin condition improved a lot after I stopped looking for a *magic* anti-wrinkle cream and listened to the needs of my skin. I am sure that no other path exists.

To have energy and a beautiful body, we need to eat right and give our body the nutrition it requires. The same is true of our skin. If we want to slow down the clock, we need to know our skin and give it what it needs on a daily basis.

19. THE MYTH ABOUT OLDER WOMEN NEEDING MORE EXPENSIVE COSMETICS

I still don't understand how I could believe that choosing the contents of my creams and serums should be based on my age. At 25, I invested in expensive anti-aging creams as it seemed obvious that my skin needed expensive ingredients so I could restore what time had already damaged.

I remember looking at those complicated names of skin care products and not being able to figure out the right time to start using them. I was convinced that one shouldn't apply really potent products on younger skin because it will get used to them, and with time, when wrinkles deepen, there will be nothing left to use, no back-up plan.

In my head, everything worked according to the advertising recommendations. I knew that, as I aged, my cosmetics would become more expensive because they contained a larger number of active anti-aging substances. At 25, I was afraid to accustom my skin to unnecessary products, so I would carefully read the labels and choose what was supposedly age appropriate.

Unfortunately, I was wrong.

Now I really know that there are no magic ingredients to be afraid of when you are young. In a later chapter, we'll discuss active ingredients that have withstood the test of time and science, and you'll be pleased to see that there is no great mystery there, either.

Our skin shows us what it needs. That's the most important thing we should pay attention to.

Many young girls are afraid of retinol because they are convinced that it is meant to fight wrinkles. But if we dig deeper, we understand that we should choose products with retinoic acid when it works for the problems we have at the time.

Retinols were developed to treat acne, little scars, and blemishes. Researchers eventually noticed that they also helped get rid of fine lines. So you should look for this ingredient in your products and not wait till you are 50. Do it when you are dealing with the problems mentioned above. Let's look at this more closely.

When you are young, all you should need is a good cleanser, cream, and sunscreen. However, if you are fighting acne, blemishes, dry patches, or if your skin has lost its glow, you should examine active ingredients to help you deal with these problems, and not be stuck in your old beliefs.

Label indications that tell you an age-appropriate time to start using a product are meant for women looking for a quick fix who know nothing about their skin. They hope they don't have to dig deeper and learn. They buy the advertising description on the package hoping that the manufacturer has their best interest at heart, even though this is rarely the case.

After reading this book, you should be armed with all the knowledge you need to protect yourself from bad decisions.

20. THE MYTH ABOUT THE BENEFITS OF COSMETIC PROCEDURES

Another name for this myth is "money for cosmetologists and procedures that went down the drain."

I used to look at cosmetologists, dermatologists, and pharmacists as my saviors. I believed their every word, bought the products they recommended, and waited for improvements.

Now I have removed my rose-colored glasses. People working in this field are the same as the rest of us. It's very difficult to find a truly good specialist. Most cosmetologists have no deep knowledge and understanding of how the skin functions. They tend to work with a very limited number of products from a few manufacturers who organize training sessions, introduce new products, teach procedures, and offer how-to seminars for products and new equipment.

I have performed many procedures like that on my clients. I am also familiar with hundreds of different skin care product lines. Unfortunately, I have to reveal an unpleasant truth—most companies are not trying to solve our problems. They just want to sell their products and convince us of their effectiveness, even though their effects are usually short-lived and have no magic in them.

The standard procedure performed by a cosmetologist goes through several steps: first, a thorough face cleansing, then a procedure using some kind of acid to get rid of dead skin cells, followed by a face cleansing to remove blackheads or pimples, which will most assuredly reappear shortly thereafter. Then a client can expect a massage to activate blood flow and a mask which the manufacturer and the cosmetologist will present as particularly miraculous. Finally, the skin is nourished with a *magical* serum that has no magic whatsoever.

Even if you know nothing about skin, a facial treatment may be useful, and you will feel its effect, but it will be short-lived.

If you want to stay beautiful for a long time, you must have similar procedures a few times a week. It's very simple but effective. Instead of spending money on facial treatments, you would be better off spending it on knowledge. Choose good products and use them daily, and not only when you have the time and means to treat yourself to a session with a cosmetologist.

I must also tell you a few words about dermatologists. If they are professional, they will help you when you have a problem. They will diagnose it and prescribe a medication. I know from experience that the usefulness of such visits often ends there.

When I visit a dermatologist or a cosmetologist, I have one test question. I ask if, in their opinion, nutrition influences our skin condition. If they give me a negative answer, I turn around and never come back.

Not that long ago, people believed that nutrition, well-being, and skin beauty were not related. But today, a new generation of doctors looks at a person as a whole system and, because they love their jobs, they deal with the problem not only superficially, but also deeply by trying to get at its root cause.

Lately, I have been visiting drugstores and asking pharmacists to recommend some products. None of the recommendations proved to be right. As soon as I held a product in my hands, I immediately could see its worthlessness. There is usually something else hiding behind the recommendations of pharmacists.

A few times I bought products filled with fragrances, alcohol, and false promises, but that will never happen again. I have learned to read labels, and I only want products that will give me long-term benefits. So here is the big take-away: if you have found a specialist, and his or her recommendations are significantly improving your skin, keep seeing him or her, but remember that you can have effective treatments at home at any time.

If the products you brought home are expensive, beautifully packaged, wonderfully perfumed, with a long list of ingredients you can't pronounce or understand, chances are you are in the hands of professionals focused on making money. Real benefits will be insignificant or non-existent. And don't forget my test question about nutrition. If you don't get an affirmative answer, this specialist probably holds old beliefs and doesn't see a person as a whole. And you don't have to fool yourself into thinking that healing takes time and more investment. Believe me, I know what I am talking about because I wasted tons of money on miraculous procedures, new treatments, and *magical* skin care products.

21. THE MYTH ABOUT THE BENEFITS OF FACE MASKS

I hate to admit it, but I was wrong to invest in face masks. I am not saying that masks are completely useless, but for skin care they're not as important as manufacturers claim they are.

Frankly, I am not quite sure what the purpose of a mask is. Let me explain.

Masks are trendy and often promoted by influencers. That's why right before the holidays, we run around looking for expensive masks to make our skin glow. No matter how much we want to convince ourselves that a mask beautifies and brightens our skin, we have to admit that a miracle can't happen in 20 minutes, just from sitting with a sheet mask or a clay mask on our face.

In my cosmetics cabinet, you will hardly find a mask because I take care of my skin daily and nourish it with high-quality products. So how can a mask be of any help? First of all, its effects are insignificant because it is applied once or twice a week, and there is no *miraculous* mask ingredient. There are several types of masks, so let's look at them right now.

Popular sheet masks are nothing but a piece of paper or a similar material soaked in serum. The packaging or promotional material often touts seductive promises that usually sound something like: *brings back your glow, skin moisturizing mask, anti-wrinkle mask, fights acne,* and so on.

Later in this book, I'll reveal the whole truth about active skin care ingredients. But just to jump ahead a bit, I'll make one comment: after reading the label of a promising mask, you'll see that it usually contains water, glycerin, a few active ingredients, alcohol, and some fragrances or preservatives, usually nothing very impressive.

In a brightening and blemish-removing mask, you might find a drop of hyaluronan and vitamin C listed in the contents. Hyaluronan moisturizes, so your skin seems to look more beautiful.

Vitamin C helps get rid of blemishes and brightens the skin, so the manufacturer can boldly claim that the mask removes blemishes. However, if you really want to get rid of them, you need to use vitamin C, acids, and retinols for quite a long time. It took me about two full years. That's why 20 minutes with a mask on your face will not produce a miracle. That's also why I choose a good quality serum, full of reliable ingredients, and I use it twice a day.

The only benefit of sheet masks is that they allow the face to absorb moisture for a longer period of time, thus enabling one or two ingredients to penetrate deeper perhaps. But there is not much evidence to support that. Only a few studies have been carried out, so there is no need to clap your hands or start cheering.

Women with oily skin love clay or charcoal masks because they leave the skin looking a little bit better. Pores shrink as the clay draws out oil from the surface of the skin and improves its appearance for a short while. Unfortunately, the effect is not long-lasting and does not solve the deeper underlying problems.

Having said that, if you enjoy the effects of wearing a mask and like to spoil yourself with this kind of treatment, why not?

The newly popular masks containing acids are simply dead skin cell exfoliants, which have already been used in cleansers, serums, and toners. If this product promises to heal acne, you'll find listed its ingredients AHA, BHA, and lactic acid. I've been using acids for many years, trying different formulas, and I find that they are one of the best skin care discoveries.

Trendy sleep masks do not impress me. After examining their contents, I realized that these masks were just creams with a few active ingredients. When you learn more about deciphering product contents, you'll see that sleep masks use the same ingredients already contained in your moisturizing cream. It's just that this time they are disguised under a different name.

Manufacturers are very clever. If they can sell two products instead of one, why not? It's our responsibility to keep learning if we want to know how to choose wisely and to stay one step ahead of them.

22. THE MYTH ABOUT REMOVING CELLULITE

My battle against cellulite, which has lasted about 25 years, never produced any dramatic results. I regret spending so much money on massages, creams, and other forms of treatment.

I have exercised all my life. As a child, I took swimming lessons, did track and field athletics, and skied, so I was more or less in top physical shape. Unfortunately, I took a break for a while and preferred to spend time with a glass of wine and a cigarette in my hand rather than try to stay young and healthy.

By the time I was 20, I was already seeing the first signs of cellulite. I was really disheartened and tried to get rid of it for a long time. I underwent cellulite reduction procedures, spent money on creams, and stopped taking contraceptive pills. If I told you that my cellulite disappeared and my appearance has changed, I would be lying.

I remember trying to "blame" my genes, but that was a dead end because neither my grandmother nor my mother ever had or have cellulite.

Both my mother and my grandmother had beautiful hair, full shapely bosoms, and no problems with cellulite. I, however, had a flat chest, weak hair, and a pronounced susceptibility to cellulite. So, once again, I didn't win the genetic lottery.

For quite a few years now, I have been practicing a healthy lifestyle. I gave up soft drinks quite a while ago, and I don't eat cake or junk food. My lifestyle helps me feel better and maintain my beautiful skin. It doesn't really help with reducing my cellulite though.

After having tried different methods, technologies, and treatments at home and, once again, having wasted a considerable amount of money, I am finally giving up on them all. I decided to maintain my healthy eating habits, but I stopped worrying about cellulite. I am a woman, and my hormones constantly fluctuate and change. I try to balance them by eating healthy food and exercising, but all my efforts have no effect on cellulite. I just have it and that's that.

When I was expecting both of my daughters, I noticed an important hormonal change, but I realized that I shouldn't interfere with these natural processes. The best I can do is learn to love my thighs even though sometimes they make me feel uncomfortable and dissatisfied.

23. THE MYTH ABOUT SUNTANNING

What do I regret most? Not using sunscreen for many years.

Today, sunscreen products have a special place in my life and heart. I am convinced that no better anti-aging product than SPF has been created yet. It's a shame I didn't know that for so long.

I liked the sun and believed that it made my skin look more beautiful, reduced acne, and produced vitamin D. I liked it until, at 25, all the blemishes I had developed in my teenage years showed up on my face because of my time in the sun. I realized how badly I was damaging my beauty and youth. Luckily, I started protecting myself at that point, after I moved to sunny and warm California. Otherwise, I probably wouldn't have been able to heal my blemishes, and I could only dream about beautiful, youthful skin.

The sun's rays age our skin and draw the water out of it. They also destroy the collagen and elastin structure, which affects the firmness of our skin. The moment we start enjoying suntanning, our skin starts fighting it, changes color, and experiences stress. Suntanning without using SPF products was a huge mistake.

Don't make the other mistake I did. When I planned to stay indoors at home, I didn't apply SPF. Then I found out that although the shorter UVB rays don't get through windows, the longer UVA rays, which are the ones that age our skin, easily reach us through the windows of our homes, offices, and cars.

If you want to have beautiful and youthful skin, start looking for a good sunscreen product today. When you find one, use it daily, no matter what you do. If you spend a lot of time outside, apply it a few times, at least on your face and neck. I know it's not always convenient, but it's worth it! It's one of the best steps you can take to help your skin.

24. THE MYTH ABOUT LIP BALMS

Using so many lip balms wasn't smart, but dry chapped lips drove me to look for relief. Oh man! Instead of getting rid of the problem, I was aggravating it! I was so upset with the condition of my lips that I had no choice but to investigate the facts and figure out what I was doing wrong.

It turns out that one of my big mistakes was licking my lips all the time. Saliva contains acid that helps prepare food for digestion. By licking my dry lips, I was aggravating the situation because the acid was burning and drying them out. Unlike the rest of our facial skin, our lips don't have oil glands, so they are not protected or nourished in this way.

Think about it. What are the qualities of your favorite lip care products? They are scented and tasty. These two features mean that the product contains ingredients that shouldn't be there. Manufacturers include them so that we experience a brief pleasure from the fragrant lips we smell and the sweeteners we lick off of them. I was so attached to my lip balms that there was no way I could believe those scented and elegantly packaged items could be harmful.

But guess what happens next? In no time at all, we develop, if not an addiction, at least a strong attachment to our lip balms, and apply them constantly and generously.

As soon as I realized that I was caught in a vicious cycle, I got rid of all my favorite lip balms with cinnamon, chocolate, strawberries, and other delightful scents.

I understood that if I wanted beautiful, healthy lips, I had to choose products that were fragrance-free and tasteless. I should also make sure that their contents included a variety of oils, glycerin, hyaluronic acid, ceramides, or various tree oils. Most importantly, a daytime lip balm should contain an SPF filter because sunrays won't help retain moisture and preserve the softness of sensitive lips. The effect is quite the opposite: visible blemishes around lips only confirm that a good quality sunscreen is necessary for this part of the face too.

25. THE MYTH ABOUT MAGIC CREAMS

Every manufacturer of beauty products tries to stand out so we can find and choose their brand among the ocean of choices. And who knows better than they what we need? That's how marketing works. Cosmetic companies put a lot of effort into trying to convince us that their products contain the *magic* ingredient we have been waiting and searching for which, like no other, will solve our problems.

I am sure you have heard about the miraculous frozen grape extract from the south of France, which makes your face glow and wrinkles disappear, or about the rich oil from Morocco with amazing properties. The list goes on and on.

Sometimes manufacturers come up with complicated scientific jargon, supposedly reflecting sophisticated technologies developed by highly respected Swiss laboratories. They explain that this particular innovation is the answer to our most important beauty questions, if not our prayers.

The truth is much simpler. If we want to have beautiful youthful skin, we have to choose appropriate ingredients and work hard to make sure we maintain our good practices and preserve our youthfulness for years to come. Beware not to fall into a carefully crafted marketing trap. Skin care is comparable to nutrition. No matter how beneficial and packed with vitamins broccoli and spinach are, eating them alone is not enough to give us the energy or complete assortment of vitamins and nutrients we need for good health, right?

That's why it is not worth believing in one cream and patiently waiting for the moment we'll become young and beautiful.

26. THE MYTH ABOUT ENDORSEMENTS

I am ashamed to admit it, but I naively believed that public reviews and endorsements or recommendations were the best proof that a product worked.

What a huge mistake! I made it so many times. And will probably make it again…

I seem to understand and can perfectly evaluate the contents of a product, as well as predict the way it works. I can understand company marketing strategies and the games they play. But once in a while, I allow myself to get tricked because my favorite YouTuber, whom I've been following for several years, caresses her skin for three minutes on the computer monitor, overjoyed with the effect of her *magic* mask containing bee propolis, aloe, and honey.

My common-sense whispers, "Ruta, you've been wrong about this so many times before. You know how much companies pay influencers to 'enjoy' products publicly. Don't buy it." But sometimes the temptation is too much.

By the time evening comes around, my mind is tired, and my first fine lines start to appear. My emotions take hold of me, and I remember my favorite influencer, Linda, caressing her glowing skin. I discreetly pay for the purchase I had decided not to make, and I wait for one more *miracle*.

If my regrettable story helps you resist at least half of the products you are tempted with by your favorite "Linda," I will have accomplished my purpose.

Marketing affects our subconscious. An enormous amount of effort is put into research on how to lull our better judgment to sleep, numb our vigilance, and make us click "Buy Now." It doesn't matter what we know. Sometimes it's just impossible to resist the temptation. And that's exactly why companies invest so much into advertising.

However, I am inviting you to take advantage of the knowledge in this book. It's a good collection of information to help you shorten the road to a beautiful skin without unnecessary expenses.

27. THE MYTH ABOUT EXPENSIVE INGREDIENTS

I made a big mistake when I replaced time-tested ingredients with more expensive ones without verifying their efficacy. While analyzing the subtleties of the cosmetics industry, I mistakenly thought that it was preferable to avoid certain ingredients at all costs because they accumulate in our body and destroy the balance of our hormone system and cause cancer.

Swept away by the trendy Clean Beauty movement, I fell into another trap. I thought I was being smart because I figured out that parabens, sulfates, preservatives, alcohol, mineral oils (made of petroleum), and silicones were harmful. I completely refused them because this growing movement *opened my eyes.*

I considered myself a wise woman, so I kept telling everybody which harmful ingredients to avoid. Unfortunately, I didn't even notice how I started paying much more money than before for everyday products.

The products involved in the Clean Beauty movement and similar products endorsed by naturalists are not *bad.* One very positive thing about them is that they promote competition and make manufacturers create cleaner and more effective products. But there is a money trail even behind these seemingly positive movements. Instead of believing every claim you come across, you must coldly examine the facts and make note of all the advantages and disadvantages you can.

Several companies influenced the Clean Beauty movement when they threw all their efforts into pushing some reliable ingredients out of the market so that their labels could tout phrases like *SLS free, paraben free,* and *silicone free.*

These manufacturers even managed to make us feel proud of our choices and dig deeper into our wallets to pay even more for similar products.

The Clean Beauty movement became so popular that huge retailers like Sephora marked their products with the movement sticker. Companies steered us to choose cleaner products, but if you look closer, you will see that they did it to benefit themselves, not us.

Let's take a quick look at a few ingredients. The truth about them lies somewhere in the middle.

Alcohol. All you have to know is that we shouldn't fear all of the alcohols in the cosmetics industry. Not all alcohols are monsters that dry our skin. Some products must contain alcohol in order to work. For example, a serum with salicylic acid, which penetrates our skin and destroys acne bacteria, needs alcohol to remove the layer of oil and open the pores.

Skin-drying alcohols are usually one of the following: alcohol, ethanol, denatured alcohol, propanol, ethyl alcohol, isopropyl alcohol, isopropanol, SD-40, and SD-39 (specially denatured).

The skin care products that contain helpful fatty alcohols that don't have negative side effects, rather than harmful ones, have the following names: cetyl alcohol, cetearyl alcohol, stearyl alcohol, myristyl alcohol, lauryl alcohol, behenyl alcohol.

Parabens. Paraben opponents all whistle the same tune: these are preservatives used in cosmetics to extend their shelf life. They are beneficial for the manufacturer, but they are harmful for consumers because they accumulate in the body and cause diseases.

However, scientific studies carried out over many years show that parabens can be beneficial for us as well. They slow down bacteria growth in creams, serums, and other products we use. They have neither the hormone-destroying nor allergy-causing effects. Of course, there are companies misusing the allowed amounts of parabens, but it's been proven that small amounts of paraben can be effective and well tolerated by the skin.

After learning that, I admitted that I certainly didn't want creams incubating large amounts of bacteria.

Silicones. A lot of bad things are said about silicones, but the facts show that not all of them are bad. Some of them are useful to us because they help *lock* moisture in our skin. If your skin is oily and you don't want moisturizers containing oils, silicones could be a good alternative.

They are effective not only for healing scars but also for baby creams that protect delicate skin from diaper rash. They also help in the application of creams by allowing for a better distribution on the skin, and they leave a more pleasant feeling.

I personally love products with silicone because my skin is not smooth. It has lots of texture because of visible pores, tiny scars, and uneven patches. That's why I don't avoid silicones in the morning. Not only do they lock in moisture in my oily skin, but they help with the even application of makeup. However, I try not to overuse them. If my cream contains silicones, I try to make sure that my SPF products or makeup foundation don't have them.

I limit the silicones in my morning beauty routine to two products; otherwise, they start clogging my pores, and I don't like the feeling I am left with. By the way, products with a lot of silicones are difficult to remove in the evening.

We shouldn't be afraid of silicones, but it's wise to control the amount we use. They are not equally good for all types of skin, but we needn't be unduly afraid of them or avoid them completely.

Mineral oils. At one point I swore I would never use mineral oils because they are petroleum products. With time I learned that I don't need to avoid them.

They are actually good for sensitive skin. There is not a single study that I could find proving the harmfulness of mineral oils. I have a suspicion that naturalists blew them out of proportion, and, as a result, we buy more expensive substitutions.

A word of warning: not every type of skin can tolerate this ingredient. If skin is very oily, mineral oil can clog the pores, but it may be perfect for dry skin. Mineral oil locks in moisture and is much more beneficial for our skin than many skin-irritating natural substitutions.

SLS (sodium lauryl sulfate). I keep changing my mind about this ingredient. From what I know, cheap foaming agents are not bad, but used in large quantities they *eat away* the protective layer of the skin and dry it out.

SLS is found in many products: facial cleansers, shampoos, body washes, shower gels, even dishwashing liquids.

Its use in cosmetics is allowed because products contain only small amounts of it, but if we calculated how many products of this type we use daily, we might change our minds. I have concluded that sulfates wash our hair thoroughly but damage its surface; therefore, I don't recommend using them very often.

I use shampoo with sulfates only when I shape my hair and only when I leave a lot of products in my hair. I do the same thing with facial products.

If I want to protect my skin from drying out, I stay away from SLS. Sometimes, when I want to cleanse my skin thoroughly, I use a cleanser containing sulfates before the procedure with acids. It helps the acid remove dead skin cells. And under no circumstances do I use SLS on my intimate parts because I have had unpleasant experiences with aggressive perfumed washes.

Essential oils. They often cause allergies, irritate skin, and cause other problems, so I avoid them and recommend you do so too.

Fragrances (both natural and synthetic) are beneficial only for the manufacturer. They help camouflage the odor of certain ingredients, and they make a product more attractive; however, they don't have any benefits for your skin.

In this chapter, you were able to learn about many products used in the beauty industry. I hope that now you will make smarter and more informed decisions when choosing products for yourself. You should be well-equipped to know if a manufacturer is trying to deceive you and empty your wallet or trying to help you. Learn this lesson, and don't let them fool you. Achieving a beautiful look is much more doable than you thought before.

And now I invite you to continue on this journey with me. Shortly you will receive valuable advice on how to cleanse your face and wash yourself. Believe me, you'll see that you had no idea about some daily secrets.

Chapter
FOUR

You can look younger if you learn to wash and cleanse your face.

WHY IT'S NOT WORTH PAYING
ATTENTION TO SKIN TYPES

The time has come to discuss the true definition of proper skin care, and to figure out where to begin if you want to enjoy your beautiful, smooth skin for years to come. Everything is much simpler than it may look at first.

The most important step is to create a skin care routine and choose the products that will help you solve your particular skin problems. However, to make the right decisions, we should discuss skin types.

In my opinion, skin type classifications are so complicated that many of us are uncertain of our actual type. In the end, we are faced with the same situation we encountered before: the classification system helps manufacturers sell a greater variety of products. It doesn't help consumers understand their actual needs.

Indicating a skin type on the label sometimes may help a buyer find their way in the sea of products. However, as soon as I learned what skin truly needs, this classification no longer made sense to me. Let me explain why.

I always thought that my skin was oily, so when I was in a store, I looked for products for oily, combination, or acne-prone skin. I purchased many skin-drying products with aggressive ingredients. My cleansers were packed with SLS. Toners contained lots of alcohol, and the creams had salicylic acid, benzoyl peroxide, and other drying ingredients. This was an outrageous amount of harsh active ingredients, which dried out my skin, making it produce even more oil than before. So you can understand why I say that I was caught in a vicious cycle.

THE FALLACY
OF SKIN TYPES

I have observed that skin goes through many changes, so it's not worth labeling it as one type or another because that complicates skin care. Our complexion is enormously influenced by the seasons and changes in the climate. Our complexion changes depending on our feminine cycle and a variety of hormonal changes like pregnancy, breastfeeding, and menopause. Our hormonal system is also affected by medication and contraceptives.

The quality of water has great influence on skin. That's why two weeks of vacation in a foreign country may drastically change your skin.

If I am stressed and lose some quality sleep, my skin immediately dries out, so I must treat it as if it's dry and sensitive.

If I use a lot of heavy makeup and strong concealers, my skin dries out even more and becomes dehydrated. The same happens if I use hot water or wash my skin too often.

In the preceding chapters, I mentioned improper skin care routines and badly chosen products, which changed my skin condition so much that I became completely confused as to the actual type of skin I had. There are so many nuances that I wouldn't advise labelling your skin as a certain type. Our skin is dynamic, so the most important task is to learn to understand its needs and then take care of them. That's why I would like to suggest a different attitude towards skin types.

Sometimes our beliefs and labeling lead us down the wrong path and prevent us from choosing wisely.

ANOTHER IMPORTANT THING TO KNOW ABOUT DETERMINING YOUR SKIN TYPE

In order to guide you, let's look at a few skin types and their features.

This is one of the most popular ways to determine skin type: cleanse your face with a gentle cleanser and towel dry it; do not apply anything on your face, and let your skin breath naturally for a while. After half an hour, go back to the mirror and carefully examine your skin.

If your forehead and nose are covered in a thin, shiny layer of oil, it probably means that your skin leans towards the oily type.

If your skin feels tight and fine lines appear under your eyes when you smile, it means your skin tends to be dry.

If your skin isn't tight and there are none of the signs just mentioned, you have won the "skin type lottery" and your skin is "normal." Another way to determine skin type is to take a careful look at its texture.

If you look in the mirror and can easily see its texture and pores, your skin is probably oily. This simply means that your pores are more active and produce more oil. Women with dry skin often have barely noticeable pores. That's why we can conclude that they have dry skin.

All skin types have their own advantages. No skin type is worse or better than another, so don't worry.

If right now you are thinking that I forgot some other important types (such as dehydrated, sensitive, or acne-prone), let me explain that these are not skin *types* but rather skin *conditions*, which we'll cover in another chapter.

When you think about it, both oily and dry skin could be sensitive and dehydrated, right? The main point I want to make here is that the skin type or age is not important, but the signals skin sends us tell us what its needs are.

Now it's time to discuss the first and most important step in skin care. I call it "Proper facial washing and cleansing."

PROPER FACIAL WASHING AND CLEANSING

Cleansing your face is one of the most important steps to master. It seems so simple—all you have to do is remove your makeup, any remaining facial products, and dirt accumulated during the day.

However, based on my experience and the experience of many women, I have discovered that very few of us know how to do it properly.

I prepared a set of important, non-negotiable rules. Knowing these rules will help you create new cleansing habits, which will help you achieve better results.

Remember what I told you earlier: there are no magic products. The most important tool is your knowledge and a couple of little tricks you will soon learn about and master. All this advice is meant for the evening skin care routine. In the mornings, it's enough to remove remaining products you applied at night, cleanse your face with water and, if necessary, use a microfiber face cloth.

Creams and serums should be applied only to wet skin, as this helps some beneficial substances penetrate deeper and more effectively. Besides, when we apply a serum or a cream on wet skin, we lock in the desired moisture and prevent it from evaporating.

A small reminder: we cleanse everything in gentle upward movements that go against gravity, of course.

THE MOST IMPORTANT THINGS YOU NEED TO KNOW ABOUT CLEANSING YOUR FACE

1. Imagination

If we want to wash and cleanse our face really well, we have to use our imagination.

I really like to imagine this picture: my skin envelops my entire body and protects my organs and blood from harmful environmental elements.

It barely lets anything in because its main job is to protect. However, it's alive and breathing; that's why its surface is covered with little holes. These little holes are the openings of little pipes leading to the deeper layers of the skin.

When cleansing our faces, we should remember that our goal is to gently remove a mix of unnecessary substances covering our skin (dirt from the environment, residual cream, makeup, and sunscreen, for example). That's why the very first cleansing should be gentle. This is what we should do: apply a little bit of cleanser on wet skin and massage it with gentle movements.

The cleanser will mix with the dirt on your face, and you should imagine how it lifts the dirt from the skin and melts it away. I'll say it again—if you want to do the right movement, you have to use your imagination. Let's imagine that our skin has many little pipes with little holes that are our pores. During the day, they collect a fair amount of dirt, and the first cleansing is meant to melt it away.

Let's not try to reduce our pores, clean them, or anything like that.

The most important thing is simply to melt away dirt and makeup.

By the way, even if you don't wear makeup every day, I hope that you still use SPF, so careful cleansing is still necessary.

2. Movements

Now let's discuss the force of movements when cleansing our face.

When I started to take care of my face, one very useful piece of advice stood out, which I want to share with you. No matter what you do to your skin, imagine that you are touching not your own face but the face of the person you love.

At no time should you ever rub it or stretch it.

Sometimes, in public pools or saunas, I see young girls and women forcefully rubbing their skin. It seems a small thing, but in reality, this behavior is a bad habit, which doesn't help our beauty with time.

Cleansing movements should be gentle and attentive. The way we touch our face with a microfiber cloth or towel should be the same.

When cleansing your face, try to feel your skin. Examine its unevenness and the areas that need your attention more, and think about why. You will be surprised to see the magic your attention and focus can do! As soon as we stop rushing through our routine and start giving our skin more attention and energy, the journey to knowing it better begins. And that is our most important goal—to pay attention and get to know our skin.

3. Time

The time we spend cleansing our face is very important. If you just rush into the bathroom and, 10 seconds later, rush out while rubbing your face with a towel, nothing good will come out of it.

I recommend you cleanse your face for about 30-60 seconds. It's enough time for the cleanser to do its job and remove all the dirt from your skin's surface.

I have noticed that if I spend less time cleansing my face, I don't give myself enough time for a gentle neckline and forehead massage. If I get carried away and take longer, my skin gets tired. You must find your happy medium and the amount of time that works best for you.

4. Double cleansing

Double cleansing is a true gift for our skin.

If you use different serums, sunscreen products, and makeup, or if you have oily and problematic facial skin, I invite you to discover the joy of double cleansing. This practice has long been recommended by dermatologists, and it's quite popular among Korean and Japanese women, who are undoubtedly the best in the field of skin care.

Let's explore what double cleansing is.

Obviously, the expression gives away that it's a facial cleansing procedure done twice. Usually, two types of cleansers are used. This method is much more effective than the usual one.

At this first step, I recommend using a microfiber cloth or a washcloth, as they help remove the cleanser as well as the dirt. If your skin is a bit drier, cleanse it with an oil-based cleanser, or a cleansing balm, milk, or lotion. These dissolve surface dirt and remove eye makeup.

Women with oily skin who use a lot of makeup may need to use a foaming cleanser and maybe even an electric brush.

If your skin is prone to acne, a cleanser with salicylic acid or benzoyl peroxide is useful at this stage. You can leave the product on your skin for a few minutes so that it penetrates deeply into your pores to destroy the bacteria lodged in them.

Then we move onto the second cleanser. At this stage, it's important to understand what your skin needs because this is the time to address its issues. We'll dig deeper into understanding its needs in later chapters.

You can use the same cleanser, but you should massage it a bit deeper into your skin.

Double cleansing is definitely a good way to start your facial skin care routine. I would like to emphasize again: your goal is not to rub and cleanse your skin until it becomes squeaky clean, but to learn about its needs and to satisfy them.

5. Water

When cleansing your face, always pay attention to the water temperature.

Choose the temperature that is the least stressful for your skin. It should neither be too hot nor too cold. Oily skin can tolerate slightly warmer water, but dry skin doesn't like the heat at all. It's important to preserve at least a minimal protective barrier to save moisture because hot water removes it very quickly and aggressively.

HOW TO CHOOSE A PROPER CLEANSER

If your skin tends to be dry, never use a soap or cleanser containing sulfates: sodium lauryl sulfate (SLS), sodium laurate sulfate (SLES), ammonium lauryl sulfate (ALS), or ammonium laurate sulfate (ALES). If I had dry skin, I also wouldn't choose products with essential oils and fragrances.

Women with dry skin can enjoy cleansing milks, balms, and oils. When taking care of dry skin, don't cleanse it in a way that destroys its protective layer, otherwise preserving moisture is difficult.

When cleansing oily skin for the second time, you can use a gel or foaming cleanser, but it must be free of harsh alkaline substances (harsh surfactants, which are hidden in the labels under the names of SLS, SLES, ALS, and ALES).

As mentioned in the previous chapter, there is presently a lot of controversy related to SLS. Many studies are currently underway, so at this point, it's not yet clear if this sulfate is harmful to our skin and hair.

Since I keep track of scientific studies and innovations, I try to avoid sulfates. If I want a foaming product, I choose milder ingredients, such as cocamidopropyl betaine.

We won't go into a thorough analysis of their contents, but I recommend you take the time to research and read about the ingredients of each of these products. It's not as difficult as it may seem initially. After analyzing about 10 cleansers, it will all become clear and understandable.

Women with oily skin usually like foaming cleansers. They leave you feeling clean, tighten your pores for a short while, and improve the appearance of your skin. However, in no time at all, your skin will start producing oil again, and the desired results will still elude you.

I suggest that you stay away from all cleansers labelled *purifying, clarifying, deep cleansing,* and so on.

For both cleansings, I use only a gentle moisturizing cleanser, which I wipe off with a microfiber cloth. In some rare cases, after I have applied heavy makeup, I use a foaming cleanser with my favorite electric facial brush.

If you are bothered by acne, you can choose any cleanser which contains AHA and BHA acids or benzoyl peroxide for your second cleansing. However, it's important to monitor your skin and moisturize it well after such a cleanse. All the ingredients that destroy bacteria and exfoliate your skin also make it really dry.

I like to see moisturizing substances in my cleansers—hyaluronic acid, ceramides, niacinamide, and so on. They will not moisturize skin by themselves very well, but they will help it maintain balance. Every facial cleansing is expected to dry out the skin, so a cleanser with moisturizing substances will be beneficial to it.

Now that we know how to cleanse the face properly, let's move on to the next important stage—solving our problems.

Chapter FIVE

The most effective, scientifically-tested ingredients
that will improve your skin condition and solve many problems,
but be careful!

N ow that you know how to cleanse your face properly, let's talk about another important step—choosing a serum or cream.

Maybe it sounds complicated, but I can promise you that after reading this chapter, it will be clear and simple.

Many companies like to confuse us in order to sell us as many products as possible, which are all supposed to solve our problems. Store shelves overflow with serums with labels that promise us smooth and glowing skin. Some other descriptions try to convince us that a particular bottle contains a *mysterious* ingredient that will make our troubles disappear.

We have already discussed most of those promises in the chapter about beauty myths. Now that you know that a miraculous ingredient doesn't exist, and as soon as you see the name of a "magic" extract on a bottle, you can react to it the same way you would to any other marketing trick trying to sell you a useless product.

If we dig deeper into the facts and actual studies, we soon see that only a few truly effective ingredients are meant for skin care, and they are time tested and proven by science. The rest of them are just theories and suppositions. Now we'll discuss a few active and really effective substances you should look for in your beauty products. We'll discuss which ingredients are really important, and why we should use them.

Let's start with the three most powerful, the superstars of skin care 101. I can guarantee that after reading this chapter, you'll embrace these *superheroes* the same way I did, and you will welcome them into your life for good!

VITAMIN A (RETINOL)

Researchers have studied vitamin A, also called retinol, very thoroughly because it has tremendous benefits.

To imagine how this substance works, let me paint a picture for you.

Think about a little particle so powerful that when it gets on your skin, not only does it start instructing your cells to regenerate themselves, but it also encourages many other processes that enhance the beauty of your skin. The faster skin produces new cells, the faster blemishes disappear, the marks left by acne become lighter and wrinkles shrink. Not bad, right?

The layer of dead skin cells (which doesn't reflect the light and gives your skin a grayish hue) becomes thinner and is replaced with new cells, so your skin begins to look fresh and radiant.

And that's not all. Retinol molecules work so hard that they perform many other functions at the same time. They tirelessly keep improving our skin condition. Retinol helps the skin produce more elastin and collagen, which are responsible for our skin's firmness and elasticity.

I could write an entire book just about retinol. But I don't want to exhaust you, so I mentioned only a few of its important qualities.

THE DARK SIDE OF VITAMIN A (RETINOL)

Of course, the relationship with retinol is more complex than it appears at first glance, and there may be a price to pay for using it because it can irritate skin. Not all skin wants to listen to these instructions, so it may start fighting back. It can become sensitive, a little flaky, or dry. It's also important to remember that retinol reacts to the sun.

Pregnant or breastfeeding women shouldn't use retinol. It's a strong substance, effectively changing the behavior of skin cells, so I recommend avoiding it during pregnancy.

You have to gradually build a friendship with this ingredient, slowly and patiently. First, choose a reliable manufacturer, and then look for the best way to include retinol into your nightly skin care routine. If your skin is dry and sensitive, I don't recommend choosing a product with a high concentration of retinol.

You must ease into it. At first, apply it onto clean and dry skin once a week. Do not mix it with any other products.

In about a month, start using it twice a week, and later, maybe three times. It depends on your goals.

If you are bothered by acne, you might look for a higher concentration and more frequent applications.

I started my friendship with retinol when I was 25. I used it to get rid of acne, blackheads, and blemishes caused by zits and the sun. Now I don't have acne, and I use retinol twice a week to maintain a faster cycle of skin regeneration.

At 42, my cell regeneration cycle has naturally slowed down, and my collagen and elastin factories take a break more often, apparently with more and more time off! With the help of vitamin A, I signal to my skin that I won't accept these changes, and that these cells have to stay as active and hard working as they were in my 20's.

However, I must warn you: when you start using vitamin A, don't expect big and rapid changes. It's a long-term friendship, and the benefits become noticeable over time.

A while ago, you could purchase retinol only with a prescription.

But things have changed, and many skin care product lines suggest even several serums with vitamin A. In my opinion, it's better to start with the ones having a lower concentration and gradually increase it.

Retinol doesn't have to be expensive or have fancy packaging to be effective. Your skin doesn't care about such things. The most important thing is a good and effective formula.

So if you are looking for a product that could really help you deal with skin problems, and you are not scared of skin flakiness or sensitivity to the sun, a serum with retinol may be a good choice for you.

But if you are looking for a product without negative side effects, keep reading. I am going to present another wonderful ingredient called vitamin B3, otherwise known as niacinamide.

EFFECTIVE, FRIENDLY, AND GENTLE NIACINAMIDE (B3)

I still can't figure out why I didn't hear about this wonderful vitamin sooner. It's rather sad. I've been interested in skin care for many years, and I've been aware of all sorts of developments, but vitamin B3 somehow slipped under my radar. This is truly a great and inexpensive science-tested substance that has noticeable effects on our skin.

Since my friendship with niacinamide is quite recent, I am trying to make up for lost time and give it a lot of attention. Its results are so compelling that it could rival vitamin A, and sometimes even surpass it.

Vitamin B3 has many positive and wonderful outcomes: it affects skin color, deals with blemishes, reduces redness and skin irritations, helps maintain skin moisture, minimizes pores, and works like an antioxidant. I also like it because it regulates oil production, minimizes pores, and refreshes the skin. The most interesting point is that it helps to heal acne and rosacea.

This ingredient doesn't have any negative side effects that I can find. It is compatible with all skin types and most cosmetic ingredients, and it's happy to take its place within your daily facial skin care routine.

I have several serums with niacinamide, and I like them all. I usually use them at night because my vitamin B3 serums are a bit thicker and stickier than what I wear in the daytime. However, when my skin gets too oily, I include niacinamide in my morning routine by adding a few drops in my day cream or SPF.

I like this ingredient so much that I look for it in different facial skin care products (SPF, cleansers, makeup base, and so on). I am happy to see that recently this ingredient has been included in many products. Importantly, make sure it's not one of the last items on the label, which would mean there is very little of it in the product.

When talking about the three most powerful vitamins, we mustn't forget vitamin C, which has had a special place in my bathroom cabinet for years.

THE WONDER OF VITAMIN C AND THE DIFFICULTY OF FINDING IT IN PRODUCTS

You have probably heard a lot about vitamin C. There's a good reason for that: it's an effective ingredient and is probably my very favorite because it's an excellent antioxidant that makes your skin glow and promotes collagen production.

First, let's discuss antioxidants.

If you want to understand the benefits of antioxidants, you must first understand free radicals. These particles were discovered in 1954 by an American bio-gerontologist named Denham Harman, who was fascinated by the process of aging and really wanted to understand it.

What we learned through his research is that our bodies constantly produce free radicals. It's impossible to avoid this process. I know it sounds rather technical, but behind these complicated terms, we find little particles that make us old and block important processes in our body and skin.

Free radicals form when our body processes food and converts it to energy. They also penetrate our bodies from the environment: pollution, cigarette smoke, and ultraviolet rays. According to the famous American physician, Dr. Joseph Mercola, free radicals are a body's natural response to toxins in our environment.

Free radicals damage our cells and destroy collagen production (the reason why our skin gets old and wrinkly). Antioxidants are the particles that fight free radicals. I often imagine the work of antioxidants as a great battle between two formidable armies. Free radicals are the *bad guys* attacking us, and antioxidants are the *good guys* defending us and killing them.

Our body and skin do a pretty good job on their own, but they appreciate any help they can get.

When we use vitamin C, we support the army of good particles, and we have more chances of winning the battle against aging. Other fantastic antioxidants include vitamin E, coenzyme Q10, retinol, and resveratrol.

I use vitamin C and I like it. I can't fully guarantee that it performs miracles because I have never used it alone, as a single ingredient over a long period of time. Having said that, when my skin starts losing its radiance, I grab vitamin C serum in my cabinet. On the days when I spend a lot of time in the sun, I apply a few layers of vitamin C serum and hope that this will help my skin deal with the sun damage.

WHAT YOU SHOULD KNOW BEFORE BUYING VITAMIN C

Now comes the bad news about Vitamin C, which makes me a little uncomfortable.

Vitamin C is recognized as one of the *powerful trio*, but there are no conclusive studies or strong scientific evidence to support this.

It's quite difficult to produce a truly effective vitamin C serum because this substance is unstable. When exposed to air and light, vitamin C turns yellow and loses its effectiveness. So when choosing vitamin C, packaging is of the utmost importance: the bottle must be opaque.

Some companies claim to have discovered certain stable forms of vitamin C that don't oxidize, but it's not yet clear if this is true, as much as we would like it to be. It could be that the vitamin C they use doesn't oxidize and is more stable, but the problem is that nobody knows if it's beneficial to the skin.

Cosmetologists often mention special forms of vitamin C, but I don't tend to believe them. They just restate what manufacturers tell them, and they certainly don't conduct further studies. So far, the most effective form of vitamin C is considered to be ascorbic acid or l-ascorbic acid. The effectiveness of all other forms is highly questionable.

Another important thing when choosing a vitamin C serum is its concentration. Its efficiency threshold seems to be at no less than 15%.

So, if you buy a vitamin C serum and see that ascorbic acid is in the second half of the contents listed on the label, it might be better to take the time to find a more effective product with a higher concentration.

Vitamin C is at its most effective when combined with vitamin E and ferulic acid.

I hope you will take the time to choose a good vitamin C serum. Look for a reliable manufacturer and don't overpay. Many companies are interested in producing a vitamin C serum to claim their share of the market, so they use a variety of tricks. To discourage buyers from returning the product because of its altered color (due to oxidation with the resultant loss of efficacy), they introduce a scented yellowish serum called citric and melon elixir.

Nevertheless, I like vitamin C serum. It's good for all skin types and can be helpful when fighting acne-caused blemishes and free radicals.

I don't want to disappoint you, but I had to mention the flip side of vitamin C. If you see a truly effective product, try it, but if it is expensive and raises doubts, just choose another serum with antioxidants, which perform similar functions on your skin.

Since skin care products are constantly changing and improving, I am not going to mention specific product names in this book. I have put all this information in a separate PDF booklet, which will be updated regularly based on product developments and technological innovations.

You can obtain the electronic booklet in PDF format by clicking on or typing:

www.chocolate4soul.com/BookReport

Chapter SIX

Secrets of skin moisturizing and the 6 best moisturizers

Today we'll discuss moisturizing your skin. After reading this chapter, you'll know what skin moisturizing really is, and which ingredients you should be looking for on the label of your moisturizing cream or serum.

I will also share with you the considerable *regret I feel about* wasting so much money, searching for the perfect moisturizer. I am writing this book with the hope that not only will it help you achieve great results and improve your skin in a short period of time, but also save you money.

In the previous chapter, we talked about active ingredients, which start to work intensely and give orders to our cells as soon as they are placed on our skin. In this chapter, we'll examine a slightly different work by different substances, which we call *moisturizing*.

Skin moisturizing is a simple action, but most women do it incorrectly. Product choices are almost limitless, but we are often unsure how to choose a proper moisturizer and when to use it. Most of us simply lack the knowledge, but we'll soon fill this gap. Perhaps, as soon as tonight your skin will be able to quench its thirst.

THE THREE STAGES OF MOISTURIZING SKIN

HUMECTANTS

This fancy word covers a group of useful ingredients that work as sponges. As soon as one of them is applied to skin, it settles in and starts screaming at the top of its lungs, "Hey, water molecules, where are you? I'm lying around just waiting for you to come!" When moisture comes, it grabs it and doesn't let it go for quite a while.

Think about this: when we moisturize our face with water, it quickly evaporates together with the water in our skin. That's why the use of humectants (think of the word *humidifier*) and moisturizers is very helpful. This water-attracting group includes hyaluronic acid, glycerin, urea, aloe, amino acids, peptides, and some other lesser known ingredients.

EMOLLIENTS

These are the agents whose main job is to soften your skin so that other substances can deeply and evenly penetrate it. When it comes to emollients, the first things that come to mind are various oils and silicones.

OCCLUSIVES

The third group of ingredients to look for in your creams is occlusives. Their job is to *lock* moisture in your skin. Often the same ingredients which soften the skin do a good job at *locking* moisture in, so it's not necessarily worth separating them. The members of this group are various oils, mineral oils, silicones, shea, waxes, and lanolin.

To summarize: the first group attracts water molecules, the second one softens the skin so that it easily accepts water and other active ingredients, and this last one makes sure that substances don't evaporate from the skin surface and have enough time to do all the good work they are famous for.

THE BEST MOISTURIZING PRODUCTS FOR YOUR SKIN

If your skin is oily, you will not like creams with waxes, shea, mineral oil, or lanolin. Skin that is lazy and doesn't produce fat needs external *fatty* help. In other words, if we don't add extra fat, all the moisture (already lacking in dry skin) will evaporate immediately. That's why dry skin cream contents often include heavy and dense ingredients which create a thick protective layer on your skin and fill the gaps between cells.

Oily skin produces more fat and can perform this task itself. It doesn't need much help to save moisture. For that reason, women with oily skin can choose only gel, lotion, or products with a similar consistency, which have more permeable softeners and moisture savers, like silicones, for example. If your skin is oily, adding more fat will not allow it to breathe and get rid of dead cells, so your pores may even get infected. That's why the serum or cream you borrowed from your friend may not suit you at all. Your skin may not need the same type of moisturizer.

All the active ingredients which will help you maintain moisture are cheap. I certainly don't recommend that you spend money on a *better* or *more luxurious* cream. It doesn't exist. There is only more expensive packaging, more expensive advertising, or some exotic ingredient (for example, a red grape extract from the South of France), which makes no difference as far as results are concerned but raises the product price. The only important thing for our skin is: does it get the elements it needs or not?

Now let's talk about truly miraculous moisturizing ingredients, for which your skin will be really grateful.

THE 6 BEST MOISTURIZING CREAMS AND SERUMS

1. Hyaluronic acid (HA).

Let's start with hyaluronic acid that was put on a pedestal many years ago.

Hyaluronic acid is a very good ingredient and is considered to be not only a moisturizer, but also an antioxidant. It belongs to the first group I mentioned—humectants. Its strongest feature is to attract water. Hyaluronic acid is relatively a new ingredient, which established its place in the beauty and wellness industry in no time at all. And for good reason—it works!

Every cosmetic product line now has a hyaluronic serum. Manufacturers try to stand out by claiming that the hyaluronic molecule in their product is special; however, it's well known that almost all cosmetic lines use different sizes of HA molecules. They all perform the same function, of course. So it's not worth paying for their "uniqueness." A couple of years ago, I bought a moisturizing serum called "Valmont" for 150 euros ($160). I still don't understand how I allowed myself to be tricked like that. Today, there is no way that I would waste my money like that, despite all of the manufacturer's *sweet talk*. The effect of hyaluronic acid lasts no longer than 24-36 hours, and its main function is to attract water to your skin. It is well-suited for all skin types.

I personally love HA serums and creams. They immediately diminish wrinkles and refresh the skin. It's nice to see how the skin, cleansed at the end of the day, rids itself of tiring elements and, like a sponge, absorbs moisture along with other beneficial substances, helping it renew itself and deal with whatever problems it may have.

That's why in my cabinet, I always have a simple hyaluronic serum without any other active ingredients. I use this serum based on my skin needs: if I spent the whole day with a thick layer of makeup on my face, and I see that my skin is tired and dried up in the evening, I don't want to give it any extra tasks like skin cell renewal and elimination, collagen production, or blemish removal.

I cleanse my skin thoroughly and carefully. I do it in two stages and for quite some time—about 7 minutes. On some days, when I have the time, I take a long shower or a bath so that my skin can get really moisturized and absorb water. Then I apply the simplest HA serum (it's very important that it doesn't contain alcohol or perfumes) and nourish my moist skin. Then I observe how my skin changes: if the serum gets absorbed very quickly, I apply another layer. I give special attention to my under-eyes. If I get distracted by something and forget to apply cream, after about 10 minutes my skin tightens up. It's a sign that water is starting to evaporate from my skin and needs to be *locked in* as soon as possible.

This won't happen on a rainy day because the air is humid, but on a hot summer day, evaporation will happen very quickly, so it's important not to forget your cream.

Remember that dry skin will need a faster and stronger *lock down*. Oily skin will produce a little bit of fat and *lock* moisture, but dry skin will not. However, it's better to be cautious and have a light cream within arm's reach to help maintain moisture.

Why I rarely use hyaluronic serums

As I mentioned, I am 42 and have many skin problems. That's why I don't want to apply an empty HA serum, which seems like a waste of time for me. I prefer HA serums that have other active ingredients— peptides, niacinamide, or other antioxidants. It's the same as nourishing your body. Sometimes all it needs is water, but if you can find fresh berries or vegetables in your fridge, why not treat it to vitamins and minerals?

You are probably wondering when it's better to use a HA serum (or any other serum which includes HA)—in the morning or in the evening? I usually perform all my skin moisturizing and nourishing routine in the evening as in the morning I don't have much time and do everything fast.

If you remember, I said that everything works the most effectively when your skin is well moisturized with water.

In the morning, I usually have only a few minutes, so I cleanse my face with water and a microfiber cloth. I then apply a light, fast-absorbing cream, to which sometimes I add a few drops of serum. As soon as the product is absorbed, I apply sunscreen and hurry to apply my makeup.

If you have found an HA serum suitable for daytime use, why not? It will moisturize your skin. My serums are usually thick, and when I apply them on my skin, they create a thick layer, which makes it difficult to apply sunscreen or makeup very well.

My attitude towards skin care is this: in the evening, we pay attention to our skin—moisturize it and deal with its problems; in the morning, we protect it from the sun and harmful environmental elements. Later I will recommend different versions of a skin care routine, so you'll be able to decide which one is best suited for your lifestyle and your needs.

A word about hyaluronic oral supplements

Oral hyaluronic supplements are very popular but, in my view, not effective. The stomach immediately breaks down HA before it has time to reach the skin.

As always, you will hear different opinions. If, however, you decide to try these supplements, I recommend that you do not spend too much money and carefully observe if there are any changes in your skin, as I still haven't found any real evidence or studies about their effectiveness.

2. Glycerin

It may be old, but this moisturizing ingredient is definitely worth paying attention to. I don't know why this happened, but somehow this wonderful and cheap ingredient became forgotten and underrated. It was probably advantageous for manufacturers to push it out of the market and replace it with something that was more expensive but not necessarily more effective.

To help you understand, and maybe even fall in love with this ingredient, think about it like this: glycerin is Cindy Crawford, Linda Evangelista, and Claudia Schiffer—the supermodels who gained fame due to their hard and painful work, and whose stories will always inspire us.

On the other hand, hyaluronic acid is like modern Instagram models Kim Kardashian or Gigi Hadid, who are gorgeous and fashionable, but have not yet stood the test of time.

Don't get me wrong, I like them all; I just wanted to give glycerin its well-deserved crown again. In case you can't tell, it is one of my favorite moisturizing ingredients.

3. Ceramides

Ceramides belong to a slightly different category. To put it simply, they are fats that fill the gaps between cells. They are especially *loved* by dry skin.

This is how I picture ceramides in my mind: I imagine them as a glue filling in the gaps in my skin and creating a fantastic protective layer so that my skin is protected from the environmental impact and loss of moisture.

Young girls and women should like products containing ceramides, as everyone's skin gets drier with time. Ceramides should also appeal to those who suffer from atopic dermatitis.

Ceramides are good ingredients but not mandatory. There are other great substances which can perform a similar function, namely urea, also known as lactic acid, and such. I like ceramides, so I look for them in the contents when selecting my cream, lip balm, or any other moisturizing product.

4. Silicones

When my skin was oilier, silicones suited it very well. At one point, they had lost their reputation—I guess someone profited from that—but now the attitude towards silicones is improving again. It was said that silicones clog pores and cause acne, but now the research and facts show something different. In my view, silicones maintain skin balance, make skin softer and smoother, protect it from negative environmental factors, and *lock in* its moisture quite effectively.

Some other vitamins which are nice to see on the label are panthenol (B5) and vitamin E. They don't have any unique properties, but they do a good job at moisturizing skin.

5. Mineral oil

For the longest time I had doubts whether it was worth using products containing mineral oil. I had read articles stating that they were made from petroleum and should be avoided. I didn't allow myself or my family members to use products containing mineral oil or paraffinum liquidum.

However, about six months ago my best friend, who has very dry skin, accidentally bought a cream whose main ingredient was mineral oil. My friend praised the newly discovered cream and insisted that it was exactly what her skin was missing for the longest time. So I decided to give mineral oil a second chance, and I began examining how and why it had gotten such a bad reputation.

I did some serious research and came across some interesting information. It turns out that mineral oil has been used in cosmetics for decades and is one of the safest ingredients to *lock in* skin moisture. That's why it's even used in baby skin care products.

Mineral oil softens skin and hair very well. It's good for sensitive skin because it doesn't have any irritating properties. It stimulates wound healing. All the warnings that it is a petroleum product causing cancer are false.

Mineral oil is a great ingredient that can not only save dry skin but is also suitable for oilier skin because it doesn't suffocate it.

After learning all of this information, I promised myself I would stop going to natural health food stores and buying expensive essential oils or scented creams and stay with products that have withstood the test of time and are based on research.

Recently, I bought a nice cheap body cream with mineral oil at the top of its list of ingredients. Now, as soon as I step out of the bathtub, I gently towel dry my body and generously apply this cream. I know that it won't let moisture evaporate, and it will create an excellent protective layer for my skin.

6. Oils

I know that women like to use all sorts of oils, so we'll discuss them a little more in the hope of figuring out if they work. We also want to know what place they should occupy in our daily skin care routine. I like my moisturizing creams to have some oils in them. They soften the skin and lock in the moisture, but I don't believe they have special powers.

In this chapter, you learned how to retain skin moisture so that your skin looks fresh, radiant, and beautiful, so I don't recommend that you rely on oils only.

Women who use oils often emphasize what they like about them: they are natural, they protect from the sun, and they work like antioxidants or moisturizers. My understanding is that oils don't fully perform any of those tasks. Oils are very different. Some of them have drying properties, which are not beneficial for our skin and hair. Oil molecules are quite big, so they just *sit* on top of your skin and create some protection, but nothing more.

Oils work well together with other moisturizing ingredients, but on their own they don't have any special benefits. For many years, I used olive, coconut, and argan oils for my skin and hair. When I didn't get the desired results, I dug deeper and learned that they don't have actual benefits. Oils should remain as ingredients in creams. Manufacturers extract their most effective components and integrate them into the product in such a way that skin gets the maximum benefit. For example, olive oil may dry out skin, but one of its compounds—squalene—is very beneficial because it softens the skin and supplements it with antioxidants. Now that we have discussed how to moisturize your skin and which ingredients are most effective for doing so, you should start looking closely at the ingredient labels on all the beauty products you buy. Now it's time to take a look at other ingredients.

INGREDIENTS TO AVOID

I was going back and forth about whether I should add one more subtopic to this chapter to remind you which ingredients you should avoid. I don't want to sound repetitive, but I feel that I must emphasize that it's better to choose scent-free serums and creams.

I also invite you to look closer to make sure that the product of your choice doesn't contain drying alcohols or essential oils, which may end up irritating your skin. Don't waste your money on a variety of trendy ingredients—caviar, gold, or silver. They are used to raise the product price, but they offer no real benefits to our skin.

On the contrary, gold and silver may have negative side effects; and when it comes to caviar, no studies were done to prove its *miraculous* effects.

Other popular ingredients you can easily get sold on are placenta, growth factors, and stem cells. No one has fully researched these substances, and their effect is not clear, so it's surely not worth wasting your money on such ingredients.

Drugstores and cosmetic stores often showcase creams with collagen and elastin, promising you'll recover your youth and skin firmness. In reality, they are not worth such praises and claims. They are considered to be average moisturizers, and the substances discussed in this chapter are more beneficial.

Chapter
SEVEN

Important rules about skin exfoliation and the most
effective products (or how to get rid of the gray)

SKIN EXFOLIATION: WHAT IS IT? WHY DO YOU NEED IT? WHAT ARE ACIDS?

Sometimes I feel that many cosmetic and medical terms are complicated for one reason only—to convince us that we should respect those professions and never allow ourselves to think that the procedures they perform are simple and can easily be done at home.

Skin exfoliation is one of those terms. It's difficult to pronounce and even more difficult to understand. Along with the word exfoliation come other complicated terms—*regeneration, pH balance, stratum corneum, epidermis,* and so on. The deeper you dig, the more complicated it becomes; you come across topics that only a chemist can understand—mixing glycol and salicylic acid, and so on.

Hearing about these topics may confuse you and make you want to cover your head. You may be concerned that playing with acids may have horrible consequences, such as burning your face or something else equally frightening. That's why we avoid products with acids and only trust specialists to perform certain procedures.

However, acids are too good to be avoided. So I will explain very clearly what skin exfoliation is all about and why it's nothing to be scared of.

This new knowledge will change your attitude, release your fears, save you a lot of money, and give you a chance to perform your daily skin care routine so professionally that you'll forget how to get to your favorite cosmetic clinic!

When I think about skin exfoliation, I remember my mother, leaning over the sink and removing all the scales from the fish my father had just caught. She wouldn't stop until she scraped off every single scale. My mother knew that if a fish is covered in a thick layer of scales, there is no point in rubbing it with spices because they will prevent the absorption of any flavor.

The same thing happens with our skin. When we are young, all the mechanisms work very well. Skin cells regenerate quickly, and skin looks fresh and radiant. Children's skin completely regenerates every twenty-eight days.

A child's body and skin are perfect, and everything works well: even if a child eats pasta, pizza, or candy, it's not a problem. Most children metabolize food very fast, they don't gain weight or develop acne, and their bodies transform pasta into complicated compounds that later become cell building materials.

With time all these processes slow down.

For our body to produce building materials, it needs quality food, controlled portions, plenty of liquids, and exercise. If we don't give it that, fat starts settling in on our thighs and waist. The body can't deal with extra food, hormones become imbalanced, and our skin becomes gray and dull. Dark and puffy under-eyes give away our indulgence in salty food we couldn't resist last night . . .

In the following chapters will talk about finding strength and motivation to eat healthier food and have a more active lifestyle, but for now, let's go back to the dead cells.

In no time at all, we'll figure out how to get rid of our skin dullness and how to recover its glow. We'll find out how to *shed those scales*, which our skin can't shed by itself because of the natural aging process or our lifestyle.

THE NEGATIVE EFFECT OF DEAD SKIN CELLS, AND WHY WE NEED TO REMOVE THEM

Skin loses its glow and appears wrinkled only because dead skin cells on its surface don't reflect light. That's why it looks gray. As soon as you find the way to remove those dead skin cells, the picture will improve rapidly.

So why should we remove dead skin cells? One reason is that active serums and creams can't penetrate those little scales and *stratum corneum*, the rough outer layer of skin, so you can't expect to fix your pigmentation, acne, fine lines, or similar problems.

But the main reason is because they can clog pores. Just imagine this: on a hot summer day your skin sweats, your pores produce fat, and dead cells *sit* on top of everything and slowly get mixed into a not-very-esthetically-pleasing pore-clogging cocktail. That's how acne, blackheads, comedones (skin-colored, small bumps frequently found on the forehead and chin of those with acne), and other "uninvited guests" appear.

I was really surprised to learn about dead skin cells. I couldn't understand why we had them to begin with. How could nature, in all its perfection, have made such a mistake and at the same time made my life so miserable?

I finally learned that there was no mistake. Dead skin cells serve their own purpose. When they settle on our skin, they create a protective layer from the sun and other environmental factors.

If we lived in the wild, we wouldn't have to worry about getting rid of dead skin cells. If we spent a lot of time in the fresh air, ate unprocessed *live* food and moved around a lot, our bodies would work perfectly, and problems like cell regeneration wouldn't bother us. If we lived in a completely natural environment, we wouldn't worry about maintaining beauty and youth. We wouldn't feel the pressure of fighting time and looking gorgeous.

But at the same time, that kind of life would have its drawbacks. We would worry about finding food, perhaps even just surviving . . . Instead of daydreaming, let's just learn how to remove dead skin cells.

THE METHODS OF REMOVING DEAD SKIN CELLS

We used to remove dead skin cells with all kinds of scrubs, brushes, towels and homemade mixes of sugar, salt, ground coffee, and honey.

It wasn't a bad way, but let's face it, it wasn't that effective. Or we used mechanical means, which did an acceptable job too.

I bruised my skin many times, scrubbed it until it was red, and spread acne all over my face. So I am very happy to use modern technologies and perform the same tasks in a more gentle and less damaging way using different types of acids.

Before I go into the use of acids and cell removal with chemical treatments, I want to emphasize that if you like mechanical scrubbing, and it gives you great results, don't give it up. Women whose skin is thick and oily often prefer aggressive skin cell removal methods. I doubt, however, whether the results they achieve are the best.

Women who have dry, thin, and sensitive skin also try to remove dead cells mechanically by using brushes and microfiber cloths. They are afraid of acids because someone convinced them that chemical cocktails would irritate their skin even more, perhaps thin it out and burn it.

There is a little bit of truth to that—if you choose a product not suited to your skin. When acids came to the market, I gave up scrubs and started using different types of acid combinations. I like how they gently and smoothly dissolve the rough outer layer of my skin (*stratum corneum*) and make it glow again.

The only mechanical dead skin cell removing device you can find in my bathroom cabinet is my electric *Clarisonic* face brush, which I use a few times a week to cleanse my pores and prevent them from collecting dirt.

CHOOSING AN ACID

First you should know that you can find acids in many different forms.

Store shelves are full of acidic products—cleansers, serums, tonics, masks, and even creams. Regardless of the form in which an acid is presented, the most important things are its potency, type, and qualities. Let's remember that we're looking for a product that will remove dead skin cells and cleanse pores.

You'll be glad to find products that work for you, because acids will solve many of your problems. They'll help you deal with acne, the little scars it may cause, and pigmentation. They will also brighten your skin, and maintain moisture, and stimulate the production of collagen, which maintains skin firmness and prevents fine lines.

A QUICK OVERVIEW OF THE MOST POPULAR ACIDS

AHA acids (*alpha-hydroxy acids*). This group of plant -and animal- derived acids is very effective and friendly, and, most importantly, it mixes well with other types of acids. The group includes glycolic acid, lactic acid, malic acid, mandelic acid, tartaric acid, and citric acid.

121

Glycolic acid is one of my favorites. Glycolic acid is a water-soluble AHA that is derived from sugar cane. It is one of the most well-known and widely used AHAs in the skin care industry. Skin easily absorbs it, and it works quickly. The stronger the concentration, the stronger the effect. I tried to figure out many times the best concentration to choose, but I never came up with a satisfying answer. The closer I looked into it, the more I came across complicated pH tables, graphics, and formulas.

It turns out that the percentage of acid concentration is not always the most important thing. The most important detail to watch for is product pH and formula.

The legal glycolic acid concentration in products used at home cannot be higher than 10%, and less than 4% is simply not effective.

And now you can forget those numbers right away because the revolutionary company "The Ordinary" produces an excellent glycolic acid with an AHA of 30%, and a BHA of 2% according to its label. And by the way, its sales have soared lately!

But let's not burden ourselves with numbers and percentages. All we need to remember is this: enter the world of acids slowly, without causing stress to your skin, trusting the chosen manufacturer, carefully observing skin reactions, and navigating the abundant supply with knowledge.

Lactic acid, or lactate, is a chemical by-product of *anaerobic respiration*, the process by which cells produce energy without oxygen around. Bacteria produce it in yogurt and our guts. Lactic acid is also in our blood, where it's deposited by muscles and red blood cells. Bottom line, it is considered gentler, so it will be more suitable for women with sensitive skin.

Malic acid is an organic compound that is made by all living organisms, contributes to the sour taste of fruits, and is often used as a food additive.

It is even gentler than lactic acid, but manufacturers don't like it very much because it's very sensitive to light, so you will rarely see it listed in product ingredients.

BHA acid (*beta hydroxy acid/salicylic acid*) is a completely different type of acid group with very different properties. AHAs are water-soluble acids made from sugary fruits. They help peel away the surface of your skin so that new, more evenly pigmented skin cells may generate and take their place. Unlike AHAs, BHAs can penetrate deeper into the pores to remove dead skin cells and excess sebum. AHA acids work at the surface, while BHA acids penetrate skin more deeply and start seriously dealing with pores—decreasing infections, destroying acne and bacteria. Furthermore, they keep working hard on the skin's surface by removing the damage caused by the sun and acne. However, BHA acid reveals its true calling and effectiveness when it gets into a pore.

BHA acid is suitable for oily, combination, and acne-prone skin. Of all of the products I have disussed, this acid really did perform a miracle on my skin.

At the moment I barely use it because it dries out my skin. At this stage of my life, I don't need to treat acne or fight blackheads and comedones, so I choose acids that work on the skin's surface (AHA group of acids). However, as soon as pimples pop up or pores clog, I open my secret cabinet and get my products with BHA or salicylic acid.

If I start feeling a certain *roughness* under the skin, I grab my BHA cleanser. If an infected zit forms, I apply an overnight product with salicylic acid, benzoyl peroxide, or sulphur.

The allowable concentration of this acid is 2%, but that is just a guiding number, not necessarily reflecting product effectiveness.

One of my favorite acid products is "The Ordinary" mask (AHA

30%, BHA 2%), an acid mix that starts working in 10 minutes. I apply it once every two weeks.

When I had acne, I adored the acid cleanser "Oda" created by a Lithuanian company.

However, the most drastic improvement happened thanks to "Paula's Choice" BHA 2% exfoliant.

I continue using "The Ordinary," "Paula's Choice," and acids of my other favorite companies, but at this point of my life, I prefer gentle overnight acid serums rather than aggressive cleansers and masks.

I don't use acid procedures recommended by cosmetologists. While studying at a beauty school in Los Angeles, I experimented quite a bit. I tested acids so strong that, after the procedure, I stayed at home for a week and applied vaseline to my peeling skin.

Weaker acids made my skin slightly flake, stronger ones made it peel, and the strongest ones made large patches of skin detach from my face!

I went through all those extreme procedures because I wanted to rid myself of the blemishes left by acne. Every time I suffered through the stinging and hiding at home, I believed that as soon as the thick layer of dead skin came off, blemishes and scars would disappear.

Unfortunately, this didn't happen. Cosmetologists recommended that I repeat the cycle of procedures or choose a stronger acid. Sometimes I would listen to them, sometimes not, but as time went by, my reflection in the mirror still saddened me.

I still don't know if those drastic procedures had any impact on the beauty of my skin. I finally grew tired of constantly peeling and healing, so I gave up on all these procedures in cosmetic clinics.

Here is the takeaway from this story: acids meant to be used by cosmetologists don't burn the skin. The most extreme effect they can have is to peel away the outer layer of your skin after about a week, when new pink skin will emerge. Products meant for use at home don't have that danger. If we use a product not as prescribed or too often, we can irritate the skin, but burn it? Definitely not.

I have enough knowledge to know that I would never again do harsh acid procedures. They are a huge stress on your skin and your wallet. My attitude towards my skin has progressively changed, and now I'm working towards my goal slowly and deliberately. I'm convinced that this type of behavior is more effective than seeking quick results, only to be disappointed in the end.

Not very long ago, my eleven-year-old daughter started developing little pimples. I saw it as a sign that her skin was asking for help to get rid of dead cells.

We chose a very light cream with a low concentration of salicylic acid. That's how we got rid of her first pimples and *chicken skin*, which formed because a dead cell layer wouldn't come off and kept a pore and a hair in it pressed underneath it.

For a month, we gently cleansed her skin with a microfiber wipe and a gentle cleanser. Every other night we applied a cream with BHA acid, and a month later my daughter's skin became so beautiful, it was difficult to remember what it looked like before we used the acid.

A word of warning for breastfeeding and pregnant women: BHA (salicylic acid) is not recommended for use due to its deep penetration into pores. If you unwittingly used it, there's no need to get stressed out. Although retinol and salicylic products are not recommended for pregnant or breastfeeding women, their harmful effects have not been proven.

THE 7 MOST IMPORTANT THINGS TO KNOW BEFORE USING ACIDS

1. Start with gentler acids

In this area, it's easy to overdo it. I remember that when I discovered acids and scrubs, and I saw what they could do for my skin, I wanted to use them as much and as often as possible. I developed an addiction.

After all kinds of procedures using acids, my skin looked better, the pores were smaller, and my face seemed brighter. Naturally, I wanted to do it again and again. I fell in the trap of abusing them, and this was a bad idea. Skin can become sensitive and irritated.

There are no specific recommendations about how often and how much to use them. This is a very individual question that depends on skin type, needs, and tolerance levels. Manufacturers usually give recommendations, but they are not necessarily the last word.

Start with lower concentrations so that your skin can slowly get used to them.

2. Protect your skin from the sun

An acid eats away dead skin cells, and the newer skin becomes exposed, so it's very easy to damage it with sunburn. If you don't have a good sunscreen you can rely on, it's better not to use acids because the harm may be greater than the benefit.

Always protect your skin from the sun when you use acids of any kind.

3. Don't mix dead skin cell removal products

Before starting to use a new acid or exfoliation method, go over your facial skin care routine and make sure that you don't have too many other dead skin cell removal products.

Women often forget or simply don't know that retinol creams, serums, benzoyl peroxide, or creams and cleansers containing urea already have cell removing qualities.

It is important not to mix dead skin cell removal products and not to use too many of these products at the same time.

4. Choose your cleanser

If you decided to start with salicylic acid, I recommend that you choose a cleanser that contains it. BHA acid is fast and effective, so at first there is no point using a harsh overnight product.

5. What to apply after using an acid mask

My recommendation is simple: after removing your mask, apply a gentle scent-free moisturizing cream.

I really love acid masks. I think that when you remove a layer of dead cells, your skin receives beneficial substances easily. After a mask, I apply several active serums. I can do this because my skin has gotten used to all types of procedures over the years, but start slow at first.

6. Always apply on clean, dry skin

If you choose an acid product that can be left on for a longer period of time, I recommend that you apply it on clean, dry skin. That way you will avoid skin irritations. More than once I have applied a long-lasting serum on a moist face; however, the long-lasting burning sensation was very unpleasant. My skin was so irritated that it was difficult to see any positive effects.

It's best to follow the manufacturer's recommendations when you use a product for the first time.

7. Don't apply to the eye or neck area

When you first start using acid products, I recommend that you avoid your neck and the area near your eye. Even if your skin is not thin and easily irritable like mine, it's better to take your time and allow your skin to get used to these products.

We have discussed several of types of acids and the main rules for using them. If you are still not clear about which acid to choose, don't worry. Let this information settle in. It takes patience and practice to get a handle on proper skin care.

In the following chapters we'll discuss skin problems. I'll recommend a variety of skin care routines, which should help you deal with your skin troubles.

Chapter EIGHT

All of your efforts to maintain beauty and youth will be worthless if you ignore this important rule.

I can't overemphasize the main rule for preserving your youth and beauty—use a sunscreen (SPF).

I learned to avoid the sun when I lived in Los Angeles. Until that point, I had no interest in this subject as it seemed irrelevant to me. After moving to California, I was forced to look into sunscreens. I had a lot of acne, and I was taking a strong medicine, so I had to stay out of the sun. I remember what a dermatologist told me after she prescribed Accutane (Roaccutane), my first acne medication. "I know that you are not going to read all the warnings you signed off on, but my obligation is to tell you this. As soon as you start taking this medicine, you must strictly avoid two things—pregnancy and the sun."

In both cases, there could have been very unpleasant consequences, so without any further delay, I went to a drugstore and bought sunscreen. I chose the strongest one I could find and started applying it the next morning.

I must admit that I didn't like SPF creams at all. They left white streaks on my skin, and my face looked oily. I couldn't find an SPF cream which allowed me to apply makeup properly, so I hated them all for many years. I was sure that all I had to do was just patiently wait till I stopped taking the medicine, and then I could forget about these products, and that's exactly what I did!

A little later another interesting thing happened . . .

I met a gorgeous girl at a Los Angeles party. She looked like a doll. Her skin was perfect—like a mix of a peach and porcelain. I couldn't take my eyes off her. I was envious of her beautiful skin because my own skin was covered in little scars and pigmentation.

We talked for a long time, and she told me that she had acted in a movie with Angelina Jolie. I couldn't stop admiring her charm. We became friends, and she offered to pick me up the next day and show me the most beautiful Malibu cafes and the best Beverly Hills stores.

I still have a vivid image of myself on that day: shorts, spaghetti straps, bleached hair in the wind. I was sitting outside trying to catch as much sun as I could while waiting for my friend.

She arrived shortly. Her body was covered with a long-sleeved shirt and thin gloves; her hair and face were hidden under a stylish straw hat and trendy sunglasses.

We walked around all day and learned quite a lot about each other. It turned out that my friend was much older than I had thought. When she told me her age, I was shocked. I started asking her about skin care and wrinkles, and she told me that the most important thing—the greatest secret for preserving her beauty and youth—was her diligent daily protection from the sun. I could hardly believe what I heard. That was it! That was the secret!

When I came home that day, my shoulders were burnt, and my face was red. But I made a big decision then and there. I wanted to have the same skin my friend had. Sunscreen had to become a part of my daily routine, and I was determined to *make it a friend* as well.

This happened about 20 years ago, and I have hardly ever stepped out into the sun without wearing sunscreen.

While living in Los Angeles, I learned to enjoy wearing white linen shirts with long sleeves, sunglasses, and straw hats. And I gave up enjoying direct sunlight on the beach once and for all.

I'm still happy about this decision and about the lesson I learned from my friend. Later, I started gathering information about skin and realized that we can do anything we want: buy potent serums, get super massages, nourish skin with the best creams, but all of these efforts will be worthless if we don't decide to protect our skin from the sun.

Sunbathing and skin treatments are two things that don't go together. It's like smoking a pack of cigarettes and going for a run to clear your lungs.

I want you to remember the story about my friend for a long time so that you start using sunscreen now. It isn't hard. In the beginning, while you're building new habits and looking for suitable products, it may be a bit of a challenge. But in no time at all, applying SPF will become as natural as brushing your teeth in the evening, and you won't notice the inconvenience.

Watching your skin become nicer and smoother is a great motivator. With time, you won't even envy your suntanned friends because you'll know for sure that in the future, they'll pay a high price for this short-term effect.

10 THINGS TO KNOW ABOUT THE SUN AND SUNSCREENS

1. The unpleasant truth

Now for the bad news.

There are many types of sunrays, but most of them are irrelevant to our discussion except for ultraviolet rays that come in two forms: UVA and UVB.

UVA rays (what we call *aging* rays) are rays that don't heat and don't burn, but penetrate more deeply into the skin, destroy cells, and play an important role in premature skin aging processes and wrinkle formation. UVA rays easily get through clouds and glass windows, so they damage our skin while we're driving in a car or working in our office sitting by the window, even on a cloudy day.

UVB rays (what we call *burning* rays) are rays that we can't see but we can feel because they give us sunburns; they literally *burn* our skin.

When these two types of rays affect our skin, cells die, the skin gets thicker and rougher, and facial contours become less defined. Being in the sun destroys collagen, which preserves skin firmness. The amount of hyaluronic acid in the skin, which is responsible for moisture, rapidly decreases. Skin becomes dry and develops fine lines.

2. Choosing a sunscreen

There are two types of sunscreen creams—mineral and synthetic. The ways they work are different. Mineral ones *create a mirror* on your skin, which reflects the sun's rays. Synthetic ones work slightly differently. They *absorb rays and transform them into heat.*

Some people prefer mineral filters because they consist of two simple substances—zinc oxide and titan dioxide. They are more natural, don't cause sensitive skin reactions, and are more suitable for children.

Unfortunately, it's more difficult to apply them, and they often leave a white layer on the skin. Synthetic filters are lighter and easier to use. Makeup applied on top of them looks nicer too.

I personally don't care what kind of filter is used. I usually choose sunscreens made in Korea because they have a perfect blend of mineral and synthetic ingredients. In general, cosmetic products made in Korea are very progressive, and I like them. In fact, I am happy to use any of their products because I know that I am getting maximum protection from the sun.

3. The meaning of SPF numbers, and why they matter

SPF (sun protection factor) numbers indicate how long you can stay in the sun without getting a sunburn. I wouldn't spend too much time thinking about minutes because every skin is unique. Here is an example:

when you apply SPF 50 and spend two hours on the beach, your face probably won't get tanned and burned. However, the bad news is that direct sunrays will penetrate the filter and age your skin anyway.

After applying an SPF 15, you won't get tanned for the first hour, but with time the sunscreen protection weakens, and your skin will start getting red or brown. If you chose an SPF 50 broad spectrum ++++ sunscreen, this means that the filter protects you from a broader spectrum of rays, and the little pluses mean that it's extra effective and therefore safer.

Sometimes I'll use an SPF 30, but only if I don't have an SPF 50 on hand.

I wouldn't recommend choosing anything higher than an SPF 50 because they are not better or more effective. I don't respect companies that sell SPF 70-100. These numbers are just advertising gimmicks meant to help sell the products for a higher price.

I usually choose SPF 8-15 for my body because I want to get tanned at least a little bit, especially get some color on my pale legs. Sometimes I don't buy sunscreen for my body because I use a self-tanning mousse and might not even even go to the beach.

If you decide to buy sunscreen, and I hope you do, I recommend that you look into products with an SPF 50.

4. When to apply sunscreen, before or after makeup?

Sunscreen should be applied after a moisturizer, but before makeup.

In the mornings after I cleanse my face, I always apply a moisturizer, wait a little bit until it gets absorbed, and after about 10 minutes, I apply my sunscreen. I dab it on very carefully, without rubbing my skin. In my mind, I picture my skin getting covered with a layer of a mirror reflecting the sun rays and protecting my skin. Then I make myself some tea and have my breakfast. After the sunscreen gets absorbed, I apply my makeup.

It's said that you can go into the sun as soon as you apply mineral filters; however, with synthetic ones you must wait about 20 minutes so that they form a protective layer.

I only apply light makeup afterwards. In the summer, I use a concealer or a foundation, which also has an SPF. I like a double layer of sunscreen. In the winter, I relax a little more and use oilier foundations, which don't always contain a sunscreen. However, I apply a product with an SPF daily, regardless of the season.

5. How long does an SPF work, and should I re-apply it?

Most skin care specialists recommend that you reapply sunscreen every two hours. If the filter is lower than 50, you probably must do it more often than that.

I don't always follow this recommendation because of my lifestyle and because I live in the city. I can't quite imagine how I can apply a layer of sunscreen on top of my makeup in-between meetings in the middle of the day.

If I spend a lot of time indoors, I don't grab my sunscreen every couple of hours. In the afternoon, when I go for a walk in the sun and feel that the sunscreen applied in the morning is not going to work, I just add another layer on top of the first. I don't care if my makeup looks bad. If I have to choose beauty or protection from the sun, I always choose the latter.

Also, I always keep a powder with an SPF in my purse and I use it on hot summer days, especially if I have to go outside, and my sunscreen was applied in the morning. It's a different story when I am on vacation.

I was afraid of getting sunburned on the hot, bright Brazilian sands, so I applied sunscreen every hour and took off my hat only for pictures.

I felt a little envious of my husband, who constantly swam and enjoyed the water. I allowed myself to take a swim only before going back to the hotel, when I knew that we would not bake for hours in the sun. It wasn't as comfortable as I would have liked, but you have to pay a price for beauty.

6. What about vitamin D?

A question that often comes up is whether we stop the production of vitamin D by applying sunscreen.

Vitamin D is very important for our bodies since it is responsible for the strength of our bones and immune system. We get most vitamin D from food or supplements. So far, I haven't found any evidence that people who love basking in the sun get more vitamin D than those who hide from it.

There was a study on people who avoided the sun and people who loved to sunbathe. Unfortunately, it didn't produce any attention-worthy results and failed to convince anyone that sun seekers have more vitamin D and are healthier.

It's not worth lying in the sun to get vitamin D. Our bodies can just as easily get it from food and supplements. I don't think that it's worth sunbathing and aging our skin when it's not clear whether this vitamin D is being produced or not.

7. Burning eyes

How can you like sunscreen if your eyes and skin start burning as soon as you apply it? This happens to some people. In order to find a suitable product, you may need to try several. One summer I ordered 6 different products until I found the right one for me.

I decided to look for a sunscreen based on respected dermatologists and cosmetologists' recommendations I found on YouTube, because last year, I learned that it's not enough just to run to the nearby drugstore.

Before choosing products, I usually read a lot about them. When choosing a sunscreen, I've examined reviews and looked for recommendations from the people who had skin similar to mine. It's important to do this homework because you will use a product daily only if you find the one that suits you.

The first sunscreen products I bought this year were too oily and some of them burned my eyes. Then I tried *oil-free* products, but I found they contained unwanted alcohols and scents, which irritated my eyes and dried out my skin, leaving it tired and oily the next day.

Then I got interested in sunscreens made in Korea. Luckily, I found a few that did not disappoint me. Not only did they not irritate my skin, but they also were made of my favorite ingredients, niacinamide and glycerin.

Buying a product you enjoy is very important. It is then essential that you apply it around your eyes and lips where the skin is sensitive and thin, and therefore needs extra protection.

If your skin is sensitive and products often burn your eyes, I recommend looking for mineral filters, which have fewer chemicals. I've noticed that with each passing year, sunscreens seem to be getting better and more pleasant overall. They don't leave the thick white layer that their predecessors did. The industry now uses nanotechnology, which enables them to create higher quality products that are also more effective.

Don't be afraid of nano details in products. They are created to lay on top of the skin and reflect the light. They can't get to our blood and damage our bodies.

I have put the names of my favorite SPF products in a separate electronic PDF booklet, which you can download at:
www.chocolate4soul.com/BookReport

8. Spray or powder?

Now let's talk about which type of sunscreen product will suit you best—a spray or a powder?

Neither.

Don't choose your sunscreen in either a spray or a powder because it's very difficult to control the amount that gets on your skin.

I have one excellent powder, which I love to use in the daytime. The only drawback is that I have to constantly guess if any of it got on my face, or am I just imagining that I am protected. I have the same feeling when I use a spray. To tell you the truth, I don't like sprays because of their contents, and unclear benefits, and the very fact that they have to be sprayed on. I don't like to inhale suspicious particles, so I guess I'm just not willing to pay that price for protecting myself from the sun.

No spray or powder can ever be an adequate substitution for a good foundation. They may not be bad and could perhaps have a place in your purse if you need something that will fit in, but I only recommend using them as a secondary sunscreen.

9. How much should an SPF cream or lotion cost?

An effective sunscreen product should cost between eight and thirty dollars, but no more than that. Of course, it all depends on the size of the container and its actual contents, but you do not need to pay a fortune for supposedly special ingredients which have a protective filter.

Sometimes manufacturers try to profit by claiming that their sunscreen products have state-of-the-art technology, and they contain a lot of antioxidants and other *magic* ingredients. I don't believe that.

After some research, I am convinced that antioxidants (Q10, vitamin C, and so on) are not effective in a sunscreen, and there is no evidence of their benefits. We should look for active and beneficial ingredients in creams and serums, but the only requirements for sunscreen are that it shouldn't irritate the skin and eyes or clog pores, but it should protect us from pigmentation and *aging* rays.

10. How much sunscreen to apply

The most recommended amount for the face is one teaspoon. It's hard to imagine what you can do with this amount on your face. It will probably be too much for one application, but you shouldn't be skimping either. I usually put a pea-size amount into my palm and use my two fingers to distribute it on my skin slowly and carefully. It's important to take your time and not to forget the undereye area, eyelids, and upper lip and neck. When the cream gets absorbed into the skin, I double-check if I have even coverage and sometimes apply an extra amount to my nose and forehead. In my opinion, it's better to apply two thin layers rather than one thick, haphazard layer.

So those are my secrets about sunscreen. Don't worry if you haven't given them much thought before. It's never too late to start. You are now better equipped to explore the fantastic products that can help you get rid of pigmentation and beautify your skin. Even if you spent half of your life adoring beaches and sunbathing, you can focus on helping your skin and protecting it going forward. Most importantly, don't procrastinate! Start your new skin care routine now.

Now that we have discussed the steps to take and the products to look for, we'll move on to the last chapter about solving our skin's problems. We'll discuss the main issues we encounter, and we'll learn how to choose products that give maximum results in a minimum amount of time and effort.

Chapter
NINE

How to solve skin problems (acne, pigmentation,
lack of radiance and firmness, and fine lines),
and become friends with sensitive, oily, or dry skin

CARING FOR PROBLEM-FREE SKIN

E ven if you don't think that you need the information in this chapter, I invite you to read it carefully. We have already discussed that every skin type needs careful cleansing, moisturizing, and sun screening. Here, we'll start with basic skin care routines. Later, we'll go beyond the basics and talk about a few ingredients that will help you deal with problems.

Let's begin our discussion with skin that is young and virtually problem-free. It doesn't have acne, dryness, or pigmentation. When I write about this kind of skin, I'm imagining my 11-year-old daughter and her friends.

Your first question might be whether you need to do anything at all. Skin like this takes care of itself, doesn't it? In my opinion, this is exactly the time to start a minimal skin care routine, which consists of cleansing your face, applying a light moisturizing or nourishing cream, and finishing off with a sunscreen.

Every morning, my daughter cleanses her face with a microfiber cloth and water. Then she applies a moisturizer, and a little later, before she goes outside, she applies sunscreen.

In the evening, I encourage her to spend a little more time to carefully remove the remaining cream on her face and the dirt that may have accumulated during the day. The first thing my daughter does is wet her face a little bit, apply a small amount of cleanser without SLS, and gently massage the skin, letting the dirt dissolve. She removes the remaining cleanser with a microfiber cloth and water. And then on the still slightly wet face, she applies a thin layer of a scent-free moisturizer that contains hyaluronic acid, ceramides, and other great ingredients that help maintain skin moisture and create a protective layer.

It's the basic skin care routine I recommend for all women who have normal, problem-free skin. My husband does the same routine because his skin is nice and smooth.

You may be wondering why we should put chemicals on our skin if it doesn't need any help. The answer is simple: at some point, when we were young, our skin was fantastic and remained that way until a certain age, when all the problems we unwittingly created in our childhood by staying in the sun and going to bed without proper cleansing started to surface.

Just think about it: in our day and age, we are living at a time when our skin is impacted by environmental factors all day long—harmful sunrays, a cocktail of car exhaust fumes and who knows what other harmful dust particles floating in the air, pollution, and smog, which end up on our skin and negatively affect it, if not outright harm it. And that's not even considering the blue light waves emitted from lightbulbs, monitors, and other devices we are constantly exposed to.

Of course, young skin can deal with all these factors, but why not give it a little help? Why not thoroughly cleanse it in the evening so that it can breathe and regenerate? Why not prevent pollution from getting into our pores, or use sunscreen in the morning, which would allow the skin to shield itself against sunrays and slow down the aging process?

Our skin gets damaged daily because it performs the very important job of protecting us and not allowing anything external into our bodies. If we want to keep it beautiful and prevent premature aging, we should give it some well-deserved help.

CARING FOR SKIN PRONE TO ACNE, BLACKHEADS, AND SIMILAR PROBLEMS

When skin starts developing acne, little black dots, those dreaded blackheads, or little bubbles underneath it, we must react to these signals because they are indicative of something else going on a deeper level. In addition to the basic skin care I just mentioned (cleansing, moisturizing, and applying sunscreen), we should add a few more steps and active ingredients that can effectively fight acne and blackheads.

Skin gets clogged for several reasons. If it's oily and pores are wide open, a lot of dirt gets lodged in there during the day. Pores may harbor a mixture of dead cells, oil, makeup, and pollution, and this mixture can become a breeding ground for bacteria. That's why you may have acne or other unpleasant skin manifestations.

Another reason that problems emerge is tired and imbalanced skin that can't shed dead cells. After sitting in a pore for a while, oil gets trapped and turns into a bubble under the skin or a wax-like blackhead.

If we want to get rid of *unwanted guests*, we have to take a few steps and choose suitable products to treat these problems. Do you remember when we talked about double-cleansing your skin? If you are dealing with one of these problems, you'll need to start implementing changes right now, and the most important one is cleansing your skin in the evening.

The first cleansing step is meant to dissolve dirt and oil, so focus on the skin's surface. For the second cleansing step, use a product that can penetrate pores and destroy bacteria. Cleansers with salicylic acid or benzoyl peroxide do the job nicely. I have always preferred products with salicylic acid because benzoyl peroxide sometimes dries out the skin.

After these steps, examine your skin closely and decide on the next product to apply. Sensitive skin probably won't want any active substances after the cleansing, so stick to a lightweight moisturizer.

Oilier skin can handle serums and creams that are rich in active ingredients. Serums with niacinamide, salicylic acid, or even retinol (retinoids) are a great option.

Remember that open blackheads and closed comedones (under skin bubbles) developed because your skin wasn't able to rid itself of dead cells. From now on, the ingredients that can do this job should become your best friends. You might want to reread the chapter about skin exfoliation and perhaps find a suitable product. It may become your favorite, once you discover the fabulous job it can do for you.

Here is a list of some of the active ingredients which have stood the test of time and have been supported by scientific evidence. Look for them on the labels of your skin care products if you want an effective treatment for acne and blackheads: AHA, glycolic acid, salicylic acid (BHA), retin (for example, retin-a), and lactic acid.

The products that quickly dry out acne usually contain salicylic acid (BHA), sulfur, or benzoyl peroxide.

Sensitive skin needs products with a lower concentration. So instead of looking for 2% salicylic acid, choose a product with 1% or 0.5% concentration. Also, look for products with azelaic acid. Instead of choosing a skin-irritating retinol, look for serums and creams with niacinamide.

Thicker and oilier skin may prefer serums and lotions with active ingredients, while thinner and more sensitive skin may prefer creams.

When my young daughter became worried about her first pimples and blackheads, we bought her some "CeraVe" cream with salicylic acid. We didn't change her cleanser because I didn't want her thin skin, which is prone to dryness, to get too many active substances. We tried to apply the cream in the evenings. Three days later, her skin developed redness and started sending signals that it didn't like something about what we were doing.

146

So we adjusted the routine: we used the active cream with salicylic acid only every other day. On the other nights, we applied a scent-free moisturizing cream from the "CeraVe" product line as well.

My daughter also sleeps on silk pillowcases, which I wash quite often. Silk has antibacterial properties and maintains skin moisture really well; when you treat acne, I strongly recommend washing pillowcases and towels more often than usual.

In the mornings, after wetting her face, we would apply some sunscreen.

In one month, all the acne and blackheads were gone, so we stopped using the cream with salicylic acid. Her skin showed us that it needed some help with getting rid of dead skin cells, so we continued to apply it just once a week.

If my skin developed acne and blackheads, I would try a more aggressive evening routine. Twice a week, I would use a cleanser with salicylic acid. A few nights a week, I would use a retinol serum, and, once a week, I would put on a *serious* acid mask. One evening—one acid. After an acid mask or cleanser, I wouldn't apply retinols (retinoids)—just a light moisturizer. On active acne, I would apply a product with sulphur, benzoyl peroxide, or salicylic acid, and leave it overnight. I would only use a moisturizing cream and sunscreen during the say so as not to exhaust my skin.

This shows you two types of skin care routines: the very easy one my daughter does, and a more aggressive one that is meant for oilier skin that's covered with acne and blackheads.

I want to give you as much information as possible about the ingredients that can help you solve the various problems we encounter over the years. I have also given you a few examples of an evening skin care routine, but you will have to do the rest of the work. To do that, you will have to examine your skin and decide where to start. My recommendation is that you start with a cleanser containing salicylic acid and, a week later, you include a stronger mask or active serum.

If the condition worsens or gets out of control, I would talk to a dermatologist and ask about stronger retinoids or antibiotics.

HOW TO REMOVE PIGMENTATION FAST

Now let's discuss something that doesn't look great on our skin, but isn't acne either. It's time to learn how to treat pigmentation, marks left by acne, and melasma (often called the *pregnancy mask* related to changes in hormones). All of these unwanted things happen to our skin because of hormonal changes, which send the instructions to produce brighter pigmentation in one part of the body or another. There was a time when my face was covered with spots of different types and colors. The ugliest ones were on my cheeks, forehead, and above the upper lip. Some of them developed from staying in the sun, others were left by acne, but the biggest patch on my forehead was *a gift* to me from my pregnancy. The good news is that I got rid of almost all of my spots and little scars, so I'm living proof that it's possible.

If we want to treat this problem, first we have to figure out how it arises.

HOW PIGMENTATION DEVELOPS

The color of our skin, hair, and eyes are determined by melanin. This word describes a whole group of pigments that are responsible for colors in live organisms.

At every second, a multitude of very interesting processes are taking place in our skin. Hormones, which have a special status in our bodies, tell our cells how to behave. One part of the *skin factory* produces collagen, another part boosts cell regeneration, and so on.

The *melanin-related factory* produces pigments of different colors. When sunrays reach our skin, the signal is sent to produce more pigment.

When a huge zit develops and skin gets infected, another instruction is received to fight bacteria and send a stronger army and some extra blood to the infected place, which often stays in the upper layers of skin and looks like an ugly dark spot. Sometimes hormonal instructions may be influenced by changes in our lifestyle, medicine, or even food.

4 STEPS TO TREAT PIGMENTATION

If we want to accelerate the process of getting rid of unwanted spots on our face, there are 4 important steps to follow:

1. Boost your skin regeneration with retinols (retinoids). This will increase the speed of the skin rejuvenation cycle, and dark spots will disappear more quickly. Old cells will be pushed up to the surface, and the pigment in the new ones will not be as bright.

2. Use acid to remove old skin cells by dissolving the upper layer more quickly, thus exposing the nicer, smoother skin.

3. Use active ingredients, which have the ability to reach the *melanin factory*, meet its manager, and negotiate a shorter workday. You don't intend to close the factory for good because it has many beneficial functions. Melanocytes give our skin its color. It's just that in the areas where pigmentation is stronger, there is a very active team at work, which is not only on overtime but on overdrive. It just gets so carried away by its enthusiasm that it forgets to stop.
   At the end of this chapter, we'll discuss the most active and effective substances.

4. Promise yourself to always use a sunscreen and stick to it no matter what. This step is the most important one. You can use the most effective ingredients, but if you don't protect yourself from the sun, your skin will be constantly getting the signal to produce more pigment: the blemishes will become even brighter instead of fading away.

GETTING RID OF BLEMISHES

How long does it take to get rid of blemishes? This depends on your determination, the effectiveness and strength of the products you use, and the size and depth of the blemishes. Some spots left by acne will beome lighter in just two weeks if you use the most appropriate products. However, the brightest and the largest spots may take a few years.

But please don't be disappointed in hearing this or be afraid that you will never see the light at the end of the tunnel. I remember what it was like when I was treating my own largest scars and blemishes. It wasn't like I was just patiently waiting for them to go away. Blemishes slowly get lighter, become less annoying and apparent, and gradually disappear. Not that long ago, I was wondering what happened to a blemish above my lip. I can't remember when it vanished.

The point of this example is simply to emphasize that we have to do our best when trying to achieve the results we seek. However, is important to focus on other things and stop finding faults with our skin, which, by the way, never promised to be perfect forever. Especially if you did many unhealthy things to it over the years.

YOUR BEST HELPERS FOR FIGHTING PIGMENTATION

Let's discuss the ingredients which have been proven to be effective by science. In the USA and Australia, the leading medicine for pigmentation is hydroquinone. It has been considered one of the most effective blemish-healing ingredients for many years. It not only effectively lightens the skin, but also stops the production of melanin.

In the United States, you can still buy gentle hydroquinone (up to 2%), but creams with stronger concentrations (4%) are strictly controlled by dermatologists. Hydroquinone is banned in Europe, and in Lithuania it's not at all popular. However, if I had serious problems with blemishes, I would look for ways to get this product.

I used it in the past. I can't say it had a ground-breaking effect, but I liked it. While living in the United States, I remember applying it and hoping that I was using a very strong substance on my skin, which, more than any other product, would be able to deal with my personal pigment *manufacturers*.

Anyway, science has advanced since it first appeared on the market or came to the public's attention, and if you look around, you can find other great ingredients and products that work really well at lightening skin and removing pigmentation. Here are some of them:

- Retinols (retinoids)
- Different acids and their cocktails (AHA, BHA, and such)
- Vitamin C (nicely brightens the skin and reduces melanin production)
- Kojic acid
- Liquorice extract
- Niacinamide (or B3)
- Alpha Arbutin
- SPF

In this chapter, you probably noticed that, while talking about blemishes and acne, I mentioned a few of the same ingredients I had introduced you to earlier. As you continue reading, you'll discover that the same substances fight many skin problems. This information will be very useful when you start creating your own skin care routine.

We still have to discuss a couple of other skin problems, and then you will have a clear picture of what kind of plan of action to put in place to help you restore and rejuvenate your beautiful skin in no time at all.

If you can wait to start your battle with the blemishes, I recommend you add a serum with retinol to your basic routine. You should use it once a week but keep observing your skin to make sure that it doesn't get irritated or completely reject the product. And remember—retinols are always applied on dry skin.

I don't like to apply any other serum or cream on top of it because I like to preserve the active substance concentration as indicated on the label. But if I notice that my skin is *getting angry*, I might apply a moisturizing cream with no other acids a few minutes later. On other nights, I will use a serum or cream with vitamin C, which, as I mentioned before, brightens the skin and lightens blemishes.

Perhaps you are wondering whether you should apply a cream after you have used a vitamin C serum? This entirely depends on what kind of vitamin C you choose. Again, there isn't one answer. You'll have to watch your skin and see if it needs another product.

These ingredients should be enough to allow you to see changes. But if you want to include other active ingredients, look for a sunscreen that has niacinamide in its list of ingredients.

Not every skin tolerates retinoids or vitamin C. If this happens to you, don't worry. Try some arbutin acid instead. It will solve the same problems we discussed in this chapter.

Now let's talk about glow and radiance.

FROM TIRED SKIN TO GLOWING, RADIANT SKIN

Most women probably dream of having glowing and radiant skin, right? It's just that most of us never stop to think about what creates skin radiance.

Radiant and glowing skin is the one that

- Quickly rejuvenates. (The rejuvenation of older skin is very slow. That's why it may not look fresh and rosy, but a good serum or cream with retinol will fix that problem.)
- Doesn't have a thick layer of dead skin cells.
- Has enough moisture in it.
- Has good blood and lymph circulation.
- Is well protected from the sun.

Rejuvenate skin with retinols

Based on previous chapters, we can assume that by now you know how to rejuvenate your skin with retinols, right? By now, you should also know how to, with the help of different acids, remove dead skin cells so that they don't just sit on top of the skin and make it look gray. If this isn't clear, you may want to go over these subjects again.

When it comes to moisturizing your skin, let me remind you that it's very important not only to use moisturizing serums with hyaluronic acid and glycerin but also to create a protective layer, which prevents the evaporation of the skin's moisture. Oilier skin will like creams and lotions with light oils, silicones, or ceramides; women with dry skin don't have to be afraid of mineral oils (let's remember Vaseline) or shea butter and other thicker products, which act like glue by filling in gaps between cells and *locking in* moisture.

It's also very important not to forget to sleep on silk pillowcases so that moisture and active ingredients continue working on your face while you rest without soaking into the pillow.

By the way, processes that take place during the night are very important: if you still don't sleep on silk pillowcases, buy yourself some as soon as possible. When you start sleeping on silk, you'll notice that your skin and hair look much better in the morning!

As soon as you start sleeping on silk, you'll notice other results too:

- ✓ Your face will no longer have the pillow imprints that eventually cause wrinkle formation.

- ✓ Silk absorbs less moisture than cotton, so your skin will remain youthful and radiant for a long time. The serums and creams you use will stay on your skin instead of being absorbed by the fabric.

- ✓ Your hair will look smoother and nicer. It will tangle less, and in the morning, it will look better than it does when you sleep on cotton pillowcases.

- ✓ Sleeping on silk pillowcases reduces friction and loss of moisture, thus preventing hair dryness and breakage.

- ✓ Antimicrobial properties of silk will prevent the infestation of dust mites, which can irritate skin.

- ✓ Your face won't sweat, because the unique properties of silk maintain temperature balance and air circulation.

THE IMPORTANCE OF BLOOD AND LYMPH CIRCULATION FOR YOUR SKIN'S RADIANCE

You already know that, under the skin, there is a net of blood vessels which supply your skin with vitamins, oxygen, and other important elements. There is also the lymphatic system meant to collect the waste. When we don't move enough and have a poor diet, our blood and lymph systems don't work well together. It's difficult to have beautiful, radiant skin if it doesn't get enough oxygen, cell building blocks, and other important components.

You also can't expect your skin to look nice if your lymph system doesn't *take out the garbage* regularly.

I want my blood and lymph circulation system to function well, so I move around, walk, and drink a lot of water. To activate blood circulation in the facial area, I use a jade roller. It helps to clean the lymph system, activates facial muscles, and improves blood flow. Awakened skin has better blood circulation and absorbs active ingredients more effectively. That means beauty and health can begin to return to your face, and acne and blemishes disappear more rapidly.

I know I keep coming back to the daily application of a sunscreen, but it's one of the most important things you can do for your skin. Do you remember that I mentioned *glow*? I'm sure you understand that skin that is tired because of overexposure to the sun or covered in blemishes just can't look glowing and fresh.

SECRETS TO MAINTAINING THE SKIN'S FIRMNESS

So here is one more bothersome issue women face—wrinkles and fine lines! How can we make them disappear?

Let's use your imagination and powers of visualization again. Under our skin, there is the net of collagen and elastin, and the gaps are filled with hyaluronic acid. This net is like a trampoline that bounces us up if we jump on it. Or imagine a rubber band that can really hurt you if you stretch it out and let it go. That's what elasticity is.

Over the years, the under-skin trampoline starts to disintegrate; skin starts to lose its elasticity and firmness. It develops gaps and holes, which allow wrinkles to form.

The net is being destroyed not only by passing years, but also by pollution and stress. In order to completely understand what firm skin is, think of the little fine line which appears on a child's face when he smiles, and which completely disappears once he stops smiling. That's what it means to have a beautiful elastic skin.

Many 40-year-old women don't even have to smile to show the strength of their collagen net and skin elasticity because it's almost non-existent. In the areas where skin often wrinkles, there are creases (usually around the lips, along the forehead, and around eyes), which don't go away anymore.

It's almost impossible to remove deep and already formed wrinkles with skin care products, but it's definitely possible to improve their appearance.

STEPS TO MINIMIZE THE APPEARANCE OF WRINKLES AND SLOW DOWN SKIN AGING

1. Remove dead cells and speed up the skin rejuvenation process.

From the previous chapters you already know that there are many dead cells on the skin. That's why it looks older. As I mentioned before, dead skin cells don't reflect the light but instead create an impression of skin being dry, gray, and old. That's why I recommend using the acids and retinols (retinoids).

2. Moisturize skin well.

Moist and nourished skin always looks younger and nicer than dry and dehydrated.

3. Learn what steps to take and what active ingredients to use to boost collagen production and slow down the aging process.

Retinols and vitamin C are the most potent boosters of the collagen net. Other active ingredients that slow down aging and the appearance of wrinkles are antioxidants, because they catch the free radicals that interfere with collagen production. By the way, drinkable or applicable collagen won't help; there is no strong evidence to support their effectiveness. I drank collagen for many years. But after researching facts and studies, I am now convinced that it's a waste of time and money to use it in this way. Studies are done by the companies that produce the supplements, so you can't trust their "facts." Many countries throughout the world have legal loopholes regarding the production of supplements, so it's difficult to control manufacturers' labels and promises.

4. Exercising facial muscles

By no means am I recommending one or another type of facial exercises. While in Los Angeles, I did them daily for half a year, but the results were disappointing. I'm glad that I stopped when I did because stretching the skin like this may not have ended well, or certainly not with the expected or desired results.

I thought I was stopping, or at least slowing down, the signs of passing time, but all I was really doing were strange gestures and facial expressions that didn't do my skin any good. Some facial muscles became more defined, but my face lost tenderness and femininity, and my skin looked tired and irritated.

I realized that these exercises were not for me. Then I became interested in gentle Eastern massages with a jade roller, or gua sha. I really enjoy Kobido massage, which is one of the most effective techniques I've discovered.

I've examined and tried many inventions whose manufacturers promised muscle stimulation with electricity or light. When I didn't get the results I wanted, I started looking for more information and experienced the same disappointment I had when I learned about collagen supplements.

When the subject of activating or exercising facial muscles comes up, I recommend you focus on Eastern massages and the use of time-tested tools, such as my favorite jade roller or gua sha.

ENLARGED PORES AND OILY SKIN

Many women who have oily skin are annoyed by their enlarged pores. As I had oily and acne-prone skin myself, I know exactly how annoying it is to see holes on your face, which not only don't add to your beauty but also create an impression of an uneven and shiny surface.

ME AND MY GIGANTIC PORES

I used to have a magnifying mirror at home that I used for popping blackheads. Of course, in a magnifying mirror, my pores looked like huge potholes filled with oil. I wanted to reduce their size at all costs. Quite often I applied a full assortment of beauty products in my *war on pores*.

I used very strong cleansers with benzoyl peroxide, SLS, and acids. For oil removal, I used tonics with alcohol (sometimes even pure alcohol). After all that, I applied pore-minimizing masks. My favorite ones were the clay, black peel off masks, or homemade ones that came straight from the kitchen. I sincerely believed in the benefits of egg whites: before many important life events, I would apply them to my face and leave them on until my skin would get so tight, I could barely stand it.

I didn't use moisturizing or nourishing creams because that didn't make sense to me. I tried my best to make my face look matte, so I most definitely didn't want to apply any glossy cream. In my makeup cabinet, there was an entire row of pore -masking products that I used almost every day. I still remember the names of those products: *Shrink pores, Blur pores, Invisible pores. . .* Later, when I studied product contents, I re-examined many products I had been using. I had never dared to look at their product labels. In my heart I was afraid that I might get really stressed out, so I avoided further examination.

When I did finally look at the labels, I found that these products have many silicones and other skin drying substances that can be quite irritating, which I would never apply on my skin at this point. These products reduce pores and fill them in for a while. But later on, they just clog them and make them look even larger.

Before I start telling you what I did to my pores, I just want to say that not all my steps were bad. Even now I would gladly apply a good quality clay mask. I definitely wouldn't use peel-off masks or homemade egg mixes, however.

I also wouldn't use so many drying products at the same time, because they really stress out the skin. Our skin is alive. As soon as it starts getting stressed or tight, other body systems become alerted and start producing even more oil to protect the skin and improve the situation. It's like *fighting windmills*: better to give it up right away. I'll share some good advice with you that helped me reduce pores so much that they became almost invisible to me and to other people as well.

WHY SOME WOMEN HAVE LARGER PORES

Pore size is determined by several factors—genetics, age, and lifestyle.

Apparently, both of my parents had large pores and oily skin when they were young, so I shouldn't expect to have velvety peach skin with invisible pores.

Age also influences the size of pores. A pore is a little tube supported by the previously mentioned net of collagen and elastin. If your skin is firm and protected from the sun, this tube is nicely tucked in. If your skin is thin, tired, and saggy, its pores look big and relaxed.

A lifestyle is a combination of eating habits, movement and exercise, and, of course, skin care.

When you eat a lot of sugar, your body produces insulin. It can develop a variety of inflammations, and oil glands may produce more oil than they should. Similar processes happen when you drink alcohol. If you want to maintain beautiful and youthful skin for many years, read the chapter about nutrition, and follow at least some of my advice.

TIPS FOR MAKING PORES LOOK SMALLER

Now we'll discuss proper skin care for porous skin and the steps to take to make your pores look smaller.

Actually, it's impossible to permanently minimize or enlarge pores. Sometimes we have the impression that we are changing their size, but reducing the size of pores is only temporary.

5 TIPS TO MINIMIZE YOUR PORES

1. Clean and properly cared-for pores always look smaller, so let's do it right.

If our pores are not properly cleansed and cared for, they store oil, dead cells, pollution, and makeup leftovers. A pore looks bigger because all this extra content actually enlarges it. Just imagine a shopping bag hanging at the check-out counter before and after it is filled with products.

The first step is a careful and thorough face cleansing. As you know, I usually recommend a double cleansing of the face. First, we gently dissolve the oil and remaining makeup; then we get to the pores and clean them up inside. To do that, we can use a cleanser with salicylic acid (BHA), because this active ingredient can penetrate a pore very quickly and clean up oil and bacteria. After a thorough cleaning, the *tubes* are left clean and empty.

By the way, breastfeeding and pregnant women should NOT use products with BHA (salicylic acid) or retinoids (retinol).

2. Remember skin exfoliation and dead skin cell removal

Just think: the fewer dead cells you have on your skin, the fewer chances they have of reaching your pores, mixing with oils, and adding to the mix.

Dead skin cell removal is a very important part of the skin care routine. However, from experience I know that it's easy to overdo this procedure. After acidic procedures, skin looks smoother and nicer, so you may be tempted to repeat it more often. I remember how difficult it was for me not to reach for my scrubs and acid combinations in my cabinet every day. It's important to develop self-discipline and stick to the schedule you have decided on. If you don't *keep to the middle of the road* and instead remove dead cells and oils too often, your skin will get angry, and instead of making you happy, it will start producing more oil to restore balance.

I can't give you exact numbers or a winning prescription for everyone. The frequency of application often depends on the product you choose.

I can only share my experience: I have used acid masks twice a week, but when I did, I had to give up other products with vitamin C, retinol, BHA cleansers, and creams.

If you use a BHA cleanser daily, you may not need extra acid masks. If you use it every other day, you may be able to apply a cream with salicylic acid or retinol once or twice a week. Clay masks also do a good job at extracting oil and dirt from pores. The effect of clay masks is very short-lived, however, so I wouldn't recommend investing a lot of time and money in them.

But these are just guidelines. You'll have to figure out for yourself what exactly is good for *your* skin. Don't be afraid to make mistakes. The damage is not going to be that big, and sometimes we learn a lot from our mistakes.

3. Developing a long-term relationship with SPFs and sunscreen

It's difficult to hold back, but this time I won't lecture you about sunscreen. You already know it—if your skin loses firmness and doesn't support pore walls, its appearance will only get worse.

4. If your skin is oily, don't apply extra oil or moisturizer.

Don't forget to moisturize your skin daily. There are many excellent oil-free moisturizers, so look for one that's pleasant and easy to use. When you buy a cream, look for the label "non-comedogenic," even though I wouldn't fully trust this information. I've bought many products labelled *non-comedogenic, oil-free,* or *fragrance-free,* but my skin still clogged and resisted. It's good to make your choices based on your knowledge and label information, but it's even more important to pay attention to what your skin has to say about the product. If you observe carefully, it will show you if it's a worthwhile product. When you find a suitable moisturizer, your skin's appearance will improve, and your hydrated skin will balance its production of oil more effectively. You'll be surprised to see how it gets less oily, and pores will look much better than before.

5. And then there will be the off days . . .

Remember that there will be days when your pores just won't look great. It can happen when you go overboard with some products, start contraceptives, experience stress, go through ovulation, menopause, or a pregnancy, or have other life events that cause hormonal changes.

At times like this, I recommend that you temporarily set aside everything you have read about minimizing pores, and treat your skin as if you are tired and stressed out.

SENSITIVE SKIN

What should you do when your skin is sensitive and red? What should you do when it won't calm down?

This chapter is not only meant for women who constantly have trouble with sensitive skin. It will be useful to all of you: no matter what your skin condition is today, it can quickly change due to life situations or unsuitable products and become tired and irritated.

So rather than skip this section, read it carefully and thoroughly.

5 TIPS FOR SENSITIVE SKIN

1. Reduce the number of products you use

If your skin is very sensitive, or suddenly becomes sensitive, the first thing you have to do is stop exhausting it with active ingredients and find a gentler, minimal skin care routine. In other words, your skin care should consist of three basic products: a gentle face cleanser, a moisturizing cream, and a sunscreen.

But that's not all. You should look at the contents of your basic products and set aside those that contain SLS, perfumes, aromatherapy oils, and other active substances that are telling your skin what to do. It would be best if your basic product content list was as short and simple as possible.

2. Don't cleanse your face too often

Frequent cleansing changes your skin pH and stresses it out. As soon as inflammations or irritations develop on your skin, it goes to work at healing itself, and the best you can do is leave it alone as much as you can. Don't interfere!

If you cleansed your face twice a day (I know that some women with oily skin do), I recommend that you cleanse and wet your face only in the evening. And please don't use salicylic acid or other aggressive cleansers. Now is not the time.

3. Choose a simple sunscreen

Sensitive skin will prefer a mineral sunscreen. If you find a cream that contains zinc oxide, your skin will be very happy. This ingredient not only protects you from the sun but also calms your skin. Chemical filters may irritate the skin, but technology is rapidly improving, so some chemical filters may be quite good for sensitive skin.

4. Give up active ingredients

If you develop a skin sensitivity, you should give up all active ingredients immediately and not try to guess which ones caused the irritation.

From my experience, it can be extremely difficult to determine what *exactly* your skin didn't like. It's even possible that irritated skin will not tolerate substances with which it never had a problem before. We can compare it to a couple's relationship. When resentment builds up, we get angry at our partner. In moments like these, everything irritates us, and it takes some time for the situation to change.

Skin can become irritated not only because of new products or stress, but because you changed the application sequence or combination of old products, or simply that circumstances have changed. If I applied my usual acid in the morning and went outside on a sunny day, by evening, my skin would send me a message that it wasn't happy. The same would happen if I kept the acid on for too long, or if I applied it on a wet face. My skin especially doesn't like any of these procedures when my period starts.

The more you observe your skin, the better you can get along with it and have fewer problems.

The only way to help your irritated skin is to apply a moisturizing cream. It will help maintain a protective layer, which your skin is trying to create from oil and other substances. The skin does this to protect itself from environmental factors so that it can calmly focus on restoring order inside.

5. When *good ideas* become *bad ideas*

If your skin is having problems, you probably shouldn't take long baths or hot showers. Wash yourself quickly with room-temperature water, because hot water destroys the skin's protective layer that your skin desperately needs at this point.

Don't even think about *calming* your face with sunrays or the heat of a tanning bed! Forget about using ice cubes in the freezer! Don't put on any calming sheet masks! These often contain ingredients that are highly unsuitable for sensitive skin and, just like active serums, are completely unnecessary, at least at the moment.

Don't rush to organic and health food stores to consult with shop assistants about which product or oil could help you. There is no such thing. Sensitive skin prefers minimal interference rather than the introduction of new products.

Give up any idea to help your skin with brushes, devices, and any kind of mechanical action.

If you are really desperate to calm your red skin, you can use a jade roller and gently roll on it on your skin for about 5 minutes. It can't be cold, and the procedure *must* be very short.

A SPECIAL WORD FOR WOMEN
WITH SENSITIVE SKIN

To finish this topic, I would like to address women whose skin is just sensitive and doesn't like changes. You may be wondering what to do about all of those excellent ingredients that you would like to use to *stop time* or deal with other skin problems you have.

When your skin condition stabilizes, you can introduce one new ingredient at a time, but be focused and gentle. Introduce them very slowly and gradually.

You'll have to look for ingredients suitable for sensitive skin. For example, retinol or vitamin C can be adapted to irritable skin. You can also cheat a little bit by putting a drop of a new serum into the daytime cream you already use.

The ways around it definitely exist, and I'm sure you'll find them. In my opinion, there is no such thing as *bad* skin; there are only *unsuitable* skin care routines or a lack of knowledge that are easy to fix in this day and age.

In order not to disappoint women who have rosacea, I want to take a few minutes to discuss what to do when this was your prize in the genetic lottery.

ROSACEA AND ENLARGED CAPILLARIES

Rosacea can bother you just as much as acne or any other skin problem. This problem is the only one I haven't had personally, but my daughter's skin has been prone to redness since she was born. That's why I've learned the basic nuances of what this kind of skin care requires.

Read this part even if you don't have the problem, because most of the advice also applies to sensitive skin. First of all, I don't really like the name *rosacea* because it doesn't say much. Basically, rosacea is a common skin condition that causes redness and visible blood vessels to appear in the central part of the face, mostly the cheeks, nose, forehead, and chin. It may also create an uneven skin texture or produce acne or small, red spots. These signs and symptoms may flare up for weeks to months and then simply go away.

But let me be more specific about what type of skin we are talking about. Women with this type of skin are familiar with the idea of sensitivity, redness, burning, hotness, dryness, and so on.

This skin condition is considered to be genetically inherited, but don't be discouraged because these days it's possible to take excellent care of your skin and visibly improve it. Another cause of rosacea may be a thinner external skin barrier, the appearance of bacteria on the skin, or something similar.

The first step is to learn what sets off an outburst of rosacea in your body. For example, my daughter's skin doesn't like temperature changes. So in the summer, we don't use strong air conditioning in the car, and in the winter, we go outside only after we've applied a thick layer of protective cream. Her skin also doesn't like chlorine pools—trips to the sauna also end up with long-term redness.

Physical exhaustion, lack of sleep, or fatigue often worsen the skin's appearance. If you have this kind of skin, you must be disciplined and not push yourself beyond your limits.

Staying in the sun will usually *reward* your skin with the appearance of rosacea and enlarged capillaries, so I recommend giving up on sunbathing for good! It's not a loss. On the contrary, it will be a great gift to your skin. A variety of psychological factors—shame, stress, and fear—may also affect your skin condition. You just have to accept this because it's difficult to predict all kinds of life situations, and they are definitely impossible to avoid.

Hormonal changes or food—alcohol, spicy food, hot teas, and even chips—may influence your skin condition as well. That's why you have to carefully watch which life events or food products provoke these reactions.

Don't worry. Rosacea is not a disease. It's a condition we can learn to live with. All of us have to deal with something. Some of us have to fight obesity, others, thinning hair. The list of conditions is endless.

Worrying or complaining won't change anything. It's better to direct our energy and focus to actively look for solutions to our problems.

What not to do when you have rosacea

1. Don't use harsh and aggressive facial skin care products.
2. Don't trust friends' recommendations or trendy ingredients promising to solve your problems quickly.
3. Don't use hot water and products with SLS to cleanse your face. Maintain your protective skin barrier.
4. Don't use mechanical scrubs and electric skin cleaning brushes.

It might be good to read the section about the sensitive skin care again and start treating your skin lovingly and attentively.

What you *can* do with this skin condition

Having learned what provokes rosacea and what we shouldn't do, we can now go to the next level and discuss what you should do, and which products are worth your attention.

1. **Azelaic acid** should become your best friend. Your skin may tolerate BHA, but you have to introduce it very slowly.

2. **Look into SPFs** for children because most of those products are mineral, and they don't have the usual skin irritating elements.

3. **Schedule some time** to choose products that are suitable for you. It may take some time before you find the suitable retinol or vitamin C form, but you can apply different vitamin C testers. Vitamin C serum usually has a low pH that can easily irritate skin, but there are less aggressive formulas. The same advice applies to choosing retinols. Look for products that are either meant for sensitive skin or that have lower concentrations of active ingredients.

4. **Learn more** about niacinamide. It's an excellent lesser-known ingredient that can help your skin without irritating it.

5. **If you want to start using** a new ingredient, test it on your skin by applying it only on the jaw area.

Finally, I just want to add that you may want to find a dermatologist who specializes in rosacea who could examine you and guide you toward what is best for your skin. I've heard that some people have managed to minimize this problem with the help of lasers, antibiotics, metronidazole, isotretinoin, sulphur cleansers, or "Soolantra" cream. I'm afraid this is where my knowledge of rosacea ends, and I recommend you consult someone with more knowledge if you still need help.

DRY SKIN

Before we discuss dealing with dry skin, I want you to visualize something.

The outer layer of skin is called the *epidermis* and the inner layer, the *dermis*. The outer layer protects the inner layer, where all of the building processes happen. Then imagine that your inner skin, your *dermis* is a mattress made up of a variety of materials that we call collagen, elastin, and hyaluronic acid. It's covered with luxurious sheets, called *epidermis,* that protect it.

Now, the outer layer of dry skin, which is dehydrated and flaky, is like the torn and worn-out sheets that won't protect the mattress. The unprotected mattress will gradually become soiled and even start to wear out in places.

In much the same way, the outer layer of skin simply won't protect the deeper layer of skin. That's why it loses moisture easily and becomes sensitive and irritated by environmental factors.

Some people are born with dry skin, and sometimes it becomes like that over time. Why does that happen? Changes are constantly taking place in our bodies, and many of them can affect our skin condition: different hormonal changes, natural aging processes, improper skin care, and environmental factors are some of them. Skin can also dry out due to retinols, air conditioning, or the sun.

When we reach 60, we all have to learn to deal with dry skin because as skin becomes thinner through the years, oil glands become lazier and shorten their workday.

As you can see, there may be any number of reasons for skin to become dry. Before discussing what to do, I'd like you to take a few minutes to see what your skin is really like. Has it been dry for many years? Or is dryness or flakiness something new?

This is very important. If your skin has been dry for many years, and it feels dry after cleansing it, you need to make it oilier. Oil glands have become lazy, so the amount of oil they produce is not enough to create a good protective barrier. You will need to help them.

If your skin has become dry more recently, it may be that it lacks moisture. It could be that seasonal changes, stress, or new skin care products have dried it out, so your job is to give it back its moisture.

From the first part of this chapter, you learned that dry skin needs oil, and dehydrated skin needs moisture. We've also talked about how to moisturize our skin, so I'll just remind you that hyaluronic acid, glycerin, and urea are best at attracting moisture to the skin.

As for dry skin, moisture is best *locked in* by different ceramides, oils, and silicones. When you look for dry skin products, you should pay attention to creams that contain shea butter and various oils.

A few tips to care for dry skin

1. **Use only gentle cleansers and never cleanse your face with hot water.** Your skin isn't producing enough oil as it is, and it is really struggling to create a protective layer. If a cleanser with SLS and hot water removes it, your skin condition will only worsen.

2. **After cleansing your face, don't let it dry.** The more effective way to preserve and *lock in* moisture is to apply moisturizing and nourishing creams on moist skin.

3. **Avoid products with drying alcohols, fragrances, and essential oils.** Choose products that contain triglycerides, ceramides, oils, and other moisture-preserving ingredients. You shouldn't choose natural oils because it's difficult to measure their usefulness. It's better when oils are part of the ingredients in a

cream, because that's when they can maximize their benefits.

4. **If you decide to use retinols,** remember that they will dry out your skin even more, and you will have to put extra efforts into moisturizing and nourishing it.

5. **If you want to exfoliate your skin,** it's better to choose gentler and less irritating acids like glycolic or lactic acid. Please don't use harsh mechanical scrubs or brushes.

6. **Sunscreen is a must.** In the first chapters, we learned that if your skin is dry, it may not have a very thick protective layer, so sunrays will damage it more rapidly and more intensely than if your skin is oily.

7. **Sleeping on silk is a must** to preserve moisture and not damage skin.

If you follow this advice, your skin will be healthy and beautiful. Dry skin is not a problem. It can demand your attention, but if you listen to its needs and create an appropriate skin care routine, it will look nice and radiant.

THE UNDEREYE AREA

What should you do to keep your undereye area beautiful and free of puffiness, fine lines, or dark circles? I wondered for a while whether I should include a chapter about undereye care in this book.

Most skin care product manufacturers have asked a similar question: should they create an undereye cream or not? The usual answer seems to be "yes." I think that this happens for two reasons.

First of all, we have become convinced that our undereye area needs a separate product. If we don't find one in our favorite skin care product line, we would look for one somewhere else. So it's customer or market driven.

The other reason is a desire for profit. People tend to pay more for undereye creams because of the belief that their contents have some special ingredients that aren't found in face creams. Unfortunately, or perhaps fortunately, that's not the case.

No matter how much we want to believe that our undereye skin is different and needs more expensive products, it's not and it doesn't.

These days, the overall attitude about skin care is completely changing. We can thank social networks for that. We all used to believe cosmetics manufacturers and their promises, but improved access to information has increasingly convinced women that most companies have only one goal in mind—to sell us as many products as possible. They do this by to convincing us that to care for our skin effectively, we have to choose a single line of products.

As YouTube and other social media grew in popularity, unbiased opinions started pouring in from all corners. Dermatologists spoke publicly about product contents and their effectiveness, consumers shared their product reviews, and the truth started to surface.

Competition in the cosmetics industry is at an all-time high. Consumers want effective products and refuse to pay for expensive packaging. Finally, everyone is beginning to realize that skin doesn't care about packaging or advertising. And everyone is beginning to realize that good results can be achieved only with effective ingredients.

I just have to add that new product lines are being created worldwide every day, and they win their customers' appreciation by making inexpensive and effective products.

So if you still want to buy an undereye cream—by all means do so! But if you are ready to change your mind, I am about to give you a lot of information about how to improve the appearance of the area under your eyes with the products you already have.

I had all kinds of problems under my eyes. When I lived in the United States and I didn't worry about my nutrition, my eyelids were always puffy, and the dark circles under my eyes were difficult to hide. When I smiled, many fine lines would appear, which drove me crazy. I started getting them when I was only 20.

Today I'm 42 and I have fewer fine lines than ever. If I can boast for a moment, I would say that I have virtually no fine lines, and I don't intend to get them for the next ten years at least!

I'll share what I learned from researching the most common under eye problems.

DARK CIRCLES

The undereye area can have dark circles for many reasons: genetics, nutrition, fatigue, lack of sleep, unsuitable skin care products, medicine, and rubbing. I was shocked to learn that for many years, I was harming the appearance of my under-eyes by using a lash augmentation serum that damaged the whole undereye area. It turns out that it can also get puffy when you eat heavy salty food, drink too many liquids, rub your skin too often, use new products, or use products that contain perfumes. If your skin doesn't like something, it retains water or gets darker to protect itself.

Puffiness may be slightly reduced with a jade roller. You could also change your nutrition or the thickness of your pillow. For example, in the evening I sometimes eat Swiss cheese and bread, but I have to stay away from watermelon and bacon. If you see heavily puffed eyelids in the morning, you should adjust your nightly eating habits.

To keep my neck wrinkle-free, I got used to sleeping on a thin pillow with a silk pillowcase. However, during my last pregnancy, my body and the area under my eyes didn't appreciate this habit, so water started to accumulate in my face and under my eyes. As soon as I bought a thicker pillow, the situation improved, and the puffiness disappeared. I tried using creams with caffeine, but I didn't see any real results.

If you inherited the tendency to have dark circles under your eyes, they usually start on the lower lid and climb to the upper lid, though that's not always the case. Sometimes these signs just help to determine if this problem is inherited or not. In any case, you should take action.

The undereye area can be brightened with the same ingredients that remove pigmentation—vitamin C, retinols, niacinamides, kojic acid, and the other active ingredients we discussed in the section about skin pigmentation.

And fine lines around the eyes can be removed with the same actions and substances we discussed in the chapter about wrinkles and fine lines.

The only difference between the skin on your face and under your eyes is that that skin around your eyes is much thinner, just like your neck or cleavage areas. That's why it's easier to irritate, stretch, or dry it out. We need to develop new habits and be extra gentle with those areas. Let's discuss what that tenderness should look like.

1. Gently and carefully removing eye makeup

From now on we'll remove eye makeup very gently, and we definitely won't rub the skin around our eyes. I remove eye makeup with the same products I use for the first face cleansing stage. That means I use a cream or oil cleanser, which gently but effectively dissolves mascara and eyeshadow. If I choose a foaming cleanser or salicylic acid, I avoid the area under eyes so it doesn't get dry or irritated.

2. What's good for the face is good for under the eyes[1]

Under my eyes, I apply the same serums I use for the rest of my face, but that wasn't always the case. I used to use a light hyaluronic serum. After it was absorbed, I dabbed some cream on top of it to lock in moisture.

I later did some research and realized that the only way to maintain a fresh and smooth undereye area is to apply all of the active ingredients I use on my face.

I started slowly. I applied a retinol or vitamin C serum only on top of the cream so that its concentration would dilute, and my skin would get used to active substances. I acted more boldly with antioxidants and applied them under my eyes at least once a day.

About three months later, my under-eyes were ready to accept active substances. Now I treat it the same as the rest of my face.

3. Always watch the undereye area

I stay focused and watch carefully what my undereye area looks like. After using stronger concealers, I moisturize and nourish it more, but I definitely don't go overboard with products.

Sometimes in the clogged skin under one's eyes, tiny white bubbles may appear which may require that a cosmetologist remove them. When I see almost any kind of skin irritation, I immediately stop the use of active ingredients and go back to my main cream—free of scents and other irritating substances.

4. Use sunscreen under the eyes all year round

I've noticed that if I am in a rush, my undereye area or some small

---

1 I was surprised to find out that undereye creams have fewer active substances than facial skin products. I always thought it was the opposite. It turns out that most manufacturers reduce the amounts of active substances to avoid complaints about irritated skin.

patches above my lips or near my ears are often left unprotected. This is an important area, and you have to be diligent and consistent with the use of SPFs.

Now you know what to do to keep the skin under your eyes nice and hydrated for many years to come!

MORE ABOUT BODY CARE PRODUCTS[2]

The skin on your body is thicker than on your face, and it doesn't need as much attention as your face or neck. However, you should apply the information you have learned in this book when you care for the rest of the body too. That means give up cleansers, creams, and other products that have strong perfumes and contain an SLS or SLES at the beginning of their list of ingredients. If you want to moisturize your skin properly, apply a cream on the skin that's still a little damp.

If you have any problems, use active ingredients. For example, you may treat body acne with salicylic acid or benzoyl peroxide products. If you have time, you could leave them on the skin for a few minutes to allow the product to reach a deeper layer of skin. For example, *chicken skin* (*keratosis pilaris*) can be quickly healed by using a cream that contains salicylic or other acids.

For the care of your intimate parts, you should definitely give up soap or other cleansers with SLS or scented substances. Foaming sulfates not only irritate the sensitive skin of our intimate parts, but also change the pH. The area should be a little more acidic to prevent bacteria growth, so look for a cleanser with a pH less than 6.

For hand care, find a cream that contains a few more ingredients than

---

2 If you have any questions about the neck or cleavage creams, I say the same thing: you don't need different products. Skin is a live and integral organ, so it's not necessary to divide it. Of course, its thickness differs, but its structure remains similar. However, if you use mechanical scrubs for your thick skin on your knees, elbows, and feet, don't do that to your chest, neck, and face.

the standard mix of oils. You have already read what does a great job at attracting moisture to the skin—glycerin, hyaluronic acid, and urea—so buy a hand cream that lists any one of them on the label, trusting time-tested and science-tested ingredients. It's good to remember that your hands would also love to wear some sunscreen!

Moist and well-maintained lips look good on any woman, so it's time to give up the lip balms you find at the store cash registers and look for better products. Most lip care products do more harm than good and are not worth your time and attention.

Manufacturers want you to get addicted to the product and use it as much as possible, so they add scents, colors, and flavors. Did you know that a sweet chocolate-scented product makes you want to lick your lips? The acid in your saliva, which is meant to help you digest your food, gets on your lips, starts drying them out, and causes burning. It becomes a vicious circle: you lick your lips, apply the balm, lick again, apply again . . .You don't understand what's happening, but your lips are getting chapped and dry.

When looking for products meant for your lips, remember the benefits of hyaluronic acid and ceramides. Don't rush into buying scented products that contain some aloe extract with a mixture of some oils.

Good products are all around us. We just have to find them. It's a shame they're rarely placed in the most visible space on the shelf, or aren't mentioned in influencers' recommendations.

This ends the chapter about skin care. I tried to cover as much ground as possible and tried not to miss anything. If you need specific product recommendations, please download my separate e-book in PDF format that lists product names at:

www.chocolate4soul.com/BookReport

I try to avoid mentioning specific brand names and products in this book because they keep getting better, more effective, and more interesting. By the way, my secret goal is to free you from relying on recommendations by giving you enough knowledge to know what to do when you look at yourself in the mirror and pick up a cream.

Chapter TEN

5 eating habits I developed at 30, which help me maintain a healthy body and beautiful skin

If you remember, earlier in the book I confessed that for many years I didn't see my body as a whole. Many doctors told me that acne, wrinkles, and health are not related to food. For some reason, many of them liked to talk about the impact of stress. No doctors in Lithuania, another European country, or the United States asked me what I ate.

The world finally woke up, and every day we have more specialists who try to focus on the human body as a whole, with a much wider perspective in general.

I have studied nutrition, skin, and all the processes happening in our bodies for so long that most of the time, I can accurately tell what a person eats as soon as I see them.

When I studied nutrition in the United States, I immersed myself in this research for many years. While walking around a store, I would often notice people with problem skin. I would follow them and watch what food products they put in their basket. That's what convinced me that our bodies and our skin reflect our nutritional habits. It's not worth believing otherwise.

If you visit a cosmetologist or a dermatologist who believes that nutrition and skin appearance are not related, run away from such a specialist as soon as possible. Over the last ten years, serious studies have been done worldwide, and they have proven many times how strongly nutrition influences our skin.

Scientists gathered the most interesting facts about the relation between food and skin when they studied people who live in the countries where there are barely any frozen dinners, baked goods, or sugar, such as in New Guinea, Paraguay, and some other islands in the Pacific Ocean. People who live there never have acne or other skin problems that Westerners have.

I can talk a lot about my relationship with food because I've changed my eating habits many times. I went through a lot in order to understand how to eat right.

SOVIET BUCKWHEAT

In my childhood, I really loved buckwheat porridge, potato pancakes, and white bread with milk. That's what our whole family ate. For the first 16 years of my life, I had no idea that many people ate differently.

Semolina porridge, sweet curd bars, cookies, sausages, and sandwiches were my staples, and I had no intention of changing anything.

Under Soviet rule, we knew very little about the influence of food on our body or skin because we had more important things to worry about.

When I started working as a waitress on cruise ships, I became familiar with a variety of world cuisines, and for several years I tasted many different foods. It was very interesting: I had a chance to see with my own eyes that every nation has its own eating habits that often influence what people look like.

AMERICAN ABUNDANCE

Cruise ship guests could get anything they wanted, anything their hearts desired.

For breakfast they could eat not only cereal or eggs but also calamari or black caviar. Almost everything that was available to 5-star cruise ship guests was available to us as well. The ship was filled with an air of abundance. After breakfast or lunch, everything on the beautifully decorated and overflowing buffet tables either went to the employees' rooms or to the trash cans.

At the end of cruise, almost all of the passengers complained about over-eating, how much weight they had put on, and yet they still kept eating. While working on the cruise ships, I saw heavily overweight Americans for the first time in my life. It was shocking to see that they were even given special chairs in the restaurants! That's when I clearly realized that something was not right with the eating habits of this nation. That's also when I came to my first food-related conclusions and learned that beautifully displayed gourmet food can become an obsession and an addiction.

On the ship, I learned many lessons about food, but I didn't pay attention at the time. I started my modeling career ten years later. In order to become slim and squeeze myself into the tiniest clothes sizes for the photo sessions, I had to recall what I had learned on the cruise ship a decade earlier, so I dove into it.

TROUBLES AS A MODEL

It was when I started my modelling career that I heard, for the first time, comments about my being too fat. I looked for ways to shed those 13-15 pounds so my agent would stop calling me "healthy-looking."

"Pimpled" and "healthy-looking" were the words I hated the most. They caused stress and affected my self-confidence.

My weight was the most important thing, so I jumped at every opportunity to get slimmer. At that time, I didn't think about eating healthy. Maybe it was for the best because I wouldn't have been able to afford it anyway. When I lived in Hollywood, I ate at McDonald's since their food was very cheap, or I bought food at the Dollar Stores. Besides, I was sure that the only way to lose weight was just to not eat anything. Instead, I smoked a lot, drank different appetite-reducing teas, took weight-loss pills, and constantly weighed myself.

The stress of living as an illegal resident in the United States, experiencing a constant shortage of money, dealing with acne, and an uncertain future exhausted me so much that I started having all kinds of health problems.

At first, my lifestyle affected only my skin. Later, other organs started sending signals as well. My menstrual cycle became irregular, and so did my gastro-intestinal system. I started losing patches of hair, and my bathroom cabinet was filled with laxatives, stomach-calming remedies, and sleep-inducing pills.

MARRIAGE CHANGED MY EATING HABITS

Then I got married and became a legal resident in California. Everything changed for the better. My husband was a wonderful, wealthy man, ready to share his life and money with me. The first year, I had no idea what I was doing. I kept going to parties and ate everything the best Hawaii or Malibu chefs could offer. In the evenings, I took slimming pills and smoked at the gym door because I had no willpower to go in. To get rid of my dark thoughts at night, I drowned myself in wine, constantly criticized my body, and often fell asleep hating myself.

For several years I lived like that without making any changes. Slowly, I observed rich people's lives and realized that not everyone lived like I did. Some of the friends who came into my life with my new lifestyle bought food in expensive stores, followed healthy diets, had closets full of beautiful sportswear, and looked fantastic. They would meet me for lunch right after working out in gyms or meeting their personal trainers, while I met them after sitting in a cafe, where I drank coffee and smoked cigarettes non-stop.

GETTING TO KNOW THE ATKINS DIET

Another interesting thing that happened at about the same time was that my husband, whose diet was no better than mine, decided to lose 45 pounds. He read a book about the popular Atkins diet, and our refrigerator suddenly contained vegetables and steaks instead of the usual "Sprite" bottles and frozen food packages.

For several months I was forced to hear about the Atkins diet and watched the person close to me on his way to achieving his dream weight. The main thing I learned while watching this process was that you can lose weight pain-free if you give up white bread, pasta, potatoes, and cheap processed products based on flour and sugar.

We continued to go to restaurants, where my husband would order a steak or some fish with grilled broccoli. The only difference was that he would ask the waiter not to put potatoes, carrots, or any other products rich in carbohydrates on his plate. The pounds were visibly melting away, but many new problems appeared. Constipation, a lack of energy, and mood swings suddenly required a lot of effort and discipline.

THE ALLURING WORLD OF NUTRITION

I finally became interested in nutrition and decided to plunge into the world of Los Angeles diets. The sources were abundant, and all kinds of books started piling up at home. Eventually, the only topic I wanted to talk about was food.

By the way, at that point I still hadn't met a single dermatologist who told me that the appearance of my skin was related to the food I was eating.

I became fully immersed in the vast and fascinating world of nutrition. I enrolled in the sports academy, got a personal trainer's license, and later started to study healthy eating. That's when I started to value quality food and learned that food products sold in different stores aren't the same.

For about six months, I didn't notice any changes in my health or sense of well-being. I grew tired of dieting. I constantly thought about food, felt hungry, kept looking at the clock and waiting for my next meal, and secretly hated all my friends who had no acne problems or a complicated relationship with food.

Life in Los Angeles was a true roller coaster. I gained a lot of experience, broadened my mind, and set my life on a different but interesting direction. I lived there for almost 11 years, and I was crazy about that city. However, I am glad I finally left it.

THE LIGHT AT THE END OF THE TUNNEL

At 30, I became pregnant with my daughter, stopped smoking, left Los Angeles, and started a new life.

As this book is about women's youth and beauty, I won't bury you in the details of my personal life. I'll just say that my daughter became one of my strongest motivations to have a better and healthier lifestyle. I kept studying nutrition, and I began to value food from a scientific point of view. I understood pasta as carbohydrates, looked for vitamin and mineral proportions in vegetables, and learned the distinction between the olive oil group of fats and coconut oil.

I can't say that I enjoyed eating at that time though. I saw everything I put in my mouth as numbers, molecules, and tables. But I think that this stage was necessary because I had to dig really deep in order to understand how food effects our bodies.

During this time, my mother had cancer and so I had to analyze nutrition from yet another point of view as well. Over a period of about six months, I read six complicated and difficult books about the link between food and cancer diseases, and I tried as best I could to help my mother. We created different diets for her, tried veganism and opted for a variety of supplements. These efforts paid off because my mother's health has been excellent ever since. Studying nutrition was not a hobby. I did it because life threw new challenges at me. I was forced to learn more about food for many reasons, not the least of which was to help myself and others close to me feel better.

The world of nutrition is constantly changing—new diets and supplements constantly emerge. The internet is overflowing with articles about losing weight fast and choosing the proper diet.

I understand that it's not easy to choose the path most appropriate for each one of us. We want to look and feel better; however, choosing the right diet and supplements can be very confusing, because they are often just advertising tricks and promises.

It becomes even more complicated when we learn that so many opinions are contradictory. Some articles and doctors encourage you to eat fish and meat; others talk about their dangers. Where is the truth? Nobody knows. Confusion and failure exhaust us. Stress makes us stuff our faces with food and forget all our worries that way.

I think it is time for us to draw some conclusions and eliminate ineffective decisions. I want to share the pearls of wisdom about nutrition that helped me maintain my weight and beautiful skin for many years.

HOW SKIN SHOWS WHAT YOU EAT

To understand how this works, you'll have to read what happens in our bodies when we eat processed food, which is mostly made up of carbohydrates (flour and sugar). You have to comprehend the processes so that you will be able to make appropriate decisions in the future.

CARBOHYDRATES AND SUGAR

As soon as a sweet white-flour pastry gets into our body, an interesting chain of reactions is triggered. The level of sugar in our blood rises, and glycation starts; to say it simply, our cells get coated in sugar.

This means that extra glucose in our blood combines with proteins and lipids in our body. This is how I imagine the process: when sugar gets into our body, confusion sets in. Sugar can't find a place where it belongs, so it grabs hold of strong, healthy cells, makes them harder, and sucks out their life.

Remember that the skin's firmness depends on two proteins—collagen and elastin. The bad news is that sugar loves adhering to both of them more than anything else. When this happens, skin cells lose elasticity and become harder and darker. Eventually, sugar lovers' skin sags and becomes dull with visible signs of aging.

Another unpleasant thing that happens is that our body usually regulates sugar levels with the help of insulin, which affects our oil glands. When there is more oil in our pores, they can easily become inflamed, and acne starts to develop.

If you want to dig even deeper, you can explore oxidative stress and free radicals. But I won't torture you with that here.

I just want to emphasize that my goal is not to encourage you to change your nutrition radically and give up sugar entirely, but to think a bit more intentionally about how to improve your habits and situation.

HOW TO RECOGNIZE SUGAR LOVERS

Fans of sweets usually have wrinkles on their foreheads. Their skin is thinned out and dull, and their eyebrows are usually thin too. Sudden jumps of insulin create pressure in adrenal glands, which, besides other effects, are responsible for the growth of eyebrows. That's why sugar lovers rarely have thick or even eyebrows.

The skin under our eyes loses firmness and looks saggy. Face maps often explain that the digestive system is closely related to the forehead, so sugar lovers' foreheads often have pimples. Fans of pastries and pasta are often recognizable by their fuller cheeks, pigmentation, and acne in the chin area. Inflammation reactions caused by gluten show up on the face as puffiness.

MY SUGAR SINS

I have to admit that I have a favorite morning ritual, which involves coffee and chocolate. I'm not proud of it. The only reason I allow myself to indulge in them in the morning is because I am very active. I believe that over the course of the day, I will burn the sugar for energy, and it won't harm me too much. Maybe it's just my excuse because I'm not ready to give up this guilty pleasure.

There is another reason too. I kept changing my eating habits until my skin finally became smooth and absolutely clean. That's why at this time, I have no real motivation to give up anything. My skin and organs are not sending me signals to change anything.

I eat healthfully during the day, so I believe that my body can handle a little dose of sugar. It doesn't need to send me any warnings through my organs and skin. I think that my skin is aging very slowly, but I wonder how much slower it would age if I completely gave up all the pastries, pasta, sweet drinks, alcohol, and appealing cakes in the cafes . . .

Maybe one day I'll have the courage to cut them out entirely, but for now, the "70-30" rule that I use is working (I'll explain it later), and I don't need to make any new changes.

WHAT TO DO WITH FRUIT
AND VEGETABLES LOADED WITH SUGAR

Nature has organized things remarkably well. What's interesting is that natural and unprocessed food products in their original form have components that don't trigger a quick and strong glycation process.

Fiber and antioxidants in fruit and vegetables deal with glucose very well, so the processes happening in our bodies don't cause permanent damage. In reality, the glycation process happens constantly in our bodies, but food products containing processed carbohydrates and sugar speed it up so we age faster.

By the way, if my goal were to lose weight, I would give up all really sweet fruit and berries (grapes, pears, pineapples, strawberries, etc.) and certain vegetables (carrots, sweet potatoes, and beets), because they have more carbohydrates than most others.

If the information in this chapter makes you want to scream, "Hey Ruta, you only live once! Why give up delicious food because of wrinkles and acne?" I have an answer for you. When we give up cake, for example, we gain more than we lose. I regained my joy of living and my self-confidence. My skin has never been as beautiful as it is today at 42! Every day I get complimented about how smooth and radiant it is. I can assure you that I never even dared to *dream* about such a day. For most of my life, I was one of those girls who would go on dates only after dark and avoided cafes with bright lights on my face.

Another important thing you can't ignore is that skin is a truly important organ. It reflects what's happening inside your body. If your skin is saggy and covered in acne, or you have dark circles under the eyes, these are serious signals that you have to change your eating habits and lifestyle. If you don't pay attention to these signals, eventually you'll have more serious problems with your organs.

Now that we've discussed carbohydrates that destroy our beauty and youth, let's discuss a few other products that seem friendly, but can also prevent us from having healthy, radiant skin.

A WORD FOR WINE LOVERS

This short chapter may not be a favorite for wine lovers who believe that antioxidants in wine are beneficial. I don't want to argue because there is some controversy about this question. I'll just share my opinion and conclusions. Some bodies tolerate alcohol very well, others don't. There are many ongoing studies about wine and alcohol, so I think that one day we'll know more precisely how much alcohol our bodies can handle. Based on current scientific conclusions, I would say this: if you drink more than one glass a night, it's too much. All alcohol contains sugar. Of course, all wines are not equal, but they are still considered carbohydrates that travel to your blood and trigger negative processes.

How to recognize wine lovers? Their faces usually have some redness that shows up on the cheeks and in the area between the eyebrows. Other signs include enlarged eyelids, enlarged pores, and either very dry or very oily skin.

Alcohol often disrupts the sleep cycle, so skin and other cells can't properly regenerate. The skin looks tired and gray. After a large amount of alcohol has been consumed, inner organs work hard to filter the unwanted contents. They often announce their overtime by the appearance of bags or dark circles under the eyes and enlarged blood vessels.

The worst combination is sipping alcohol while lying in the sun. The sun ages your skin and destroys collagen with its UVA rays, and if you add a cocktail to that, it will coat your collagen and elastin in sugar, making them harder and less elastic.

If only you knew how hard it is for me to write these words . . . I remember countless hours spent in the pool, enjoying the hot Hawaiian sun, sipping *piña colada*s. And if I start thinking about those evening meditations with wine and cigarettes, I will beat myself up and cry.

The good news is that you can stop aging yourself at any time. After I gave up sunbathing and improved my eating habits, my skin condition improved very quickly. Even today I don't always turn down a glass of wine or some sweets, but I do it consciously and moderately.

THE IMPACT OF DAIRY PRODUCTS ON THE SKIN

I have nothing against milk, but I have met many women who improved their skin condition by giving up dairy products altogether. I have concluded that dairy products are definitely not meant for everyone. For some, it will cause inflammations and oxidative stress, which means that not only will skin age faster, but it will also develop acne.

A study performed in 2011 showed that acne is often related to hormones. Milk contains proteins and hormones that affect our body's hormones and cause acne breakouts.

Some people's bodies don't possess the enzymes necessary to process protein. If you like milk, yogurt, cottage cheese, or any kind of cheese, watch for body signals when you consume these products. Swollen eyelids, bags or dark circles under the eyes, or little white pimples on your chin may be a clear warning that you need to watch your dairy intake.

I hope I convinced you to pay at least some attention to your eating habits. No matter how good your beauty creams and serums are, if you buy sweets, snacks, pasta, or all sorts of goodies from the bakery every time you shop, you can forget about beautiful radiant skin.

There is no need to get stressed over what you eat or make drastic decisions that will be difficult to follow. There is no perfect diet. Our nutritional demands are dynamic and change constantly, but we can trust nature itself and choose the products it created for us, not the ones processed by people.

When I get lax and need the motivation to get started, I remember the *butterfly effect*. It's a beautiful metaphor about the interconnectedness of everything using a butterfly as an example: it may look very small and tender, but when it flaps its wings for a long time, it can cause a typhoon in another part of the world.

This wonderful metaphor should inspire us to take small steps and trust that eventually we'll fulfill our dreams. If you've been dreaming for a while about working out, but you don't have enough time and motivation, set yourself a small goal or an easy one—start walking every day for at least 15 minutes. I assure you that, in a week, you'll sleep better, have more energy, and even see an improvement in your mood and relationships.

Maybe for a long time you've wanted to take better care of your skin, but you think that you need more products, so you've been putting off starting your new routine. In that case, buy just one new high-quality product and watch how it changes your skin condition. The truth is that as soon as we start *flapping our wings* and taking new steps, motivation and results come naturally, without major efforts.

By making small changes that are easy for us, we won't feel stress or the need to use our willpower. It becomes simple and easy to stay on track.

Next we'll explore five habits I developed while studying nutrition and looking for food products that were good for me. I recommend you read everything very carefully because I wholeheartedly believe that our relationship with food is crucial. It lasts a lifetime. The sooner we improve it, the better we'll feel.

THE FIRST HABIT:
THE 70-30 EATING RULE

During the day, I watch what I eat and make sure that the majority of my food is beneficial for my health and beauty. I usually start my morning with eggs and vegetables, or a green smoothie of fruit and vegetables.

I don't think anyone can truly give us complete eating advice or tell us how to create a healthy personalized meal plan. Maybe in the beginning, when we make the decision to change our eating habits, having a plan might be useful, but in time, we'll feel limited, uncomfortable, deprived, and think about food all the time. It will take up a lot of space in our lives until one day we'll be so frustrated that we'll want to drop everything. If I decided to stick to one or another meal plan, I would do it only for a very short period of time. My only goal would be to examine how these products affect my mood and appearance. Later, I would pick out the best parts, include them in my daily routine, and forget about the rest.

A few years ago, my husband decided to give up sugar. He tried a program that was spread out over several months that helped him during the transitional period. It definitely wasn't easy, but he was really motivated, the program was good, and the support from the nutritional specialists was impressive. Ever since then, my husband hasn't eaten sugary cakes, candies, or baked goods with sugar.

Sometimes we attend seminars about food that is completely different from what we eat at home. These tend to be about vegetarian or vegan dishes that change our sense of well-being when we taste them. The new sensations are quite interesting, but as soon as we get home, we fall back into our usual eating habits.

WHAT WE EAT AND
WHAT MAKES UP 70% OF OUR DIET

I have several rules that I follow.

1. **My definition of good food.** For me, good food comes down to a short list: eggs, fish, meat, vegetables, fruit, and healthy fats (olive and coconut oils, avocados, and nuts). I always prefer fresh products from a market or a farm, but I buy a number of products in the supermarkets as well.

2. **Easy preparation.** I try to feed my family food that is easily prepared. Basically, all of the food we eat can be prepared quickly. I am convinced that when you boil eggs or fry or bake meat and vegetables for a long time, they change their structure and lose vitamins and minerals. It becomes difficult for our bodies to extract their beneficial components. So I think that good and useful products are those that haven't undergone a long thermal processing.

For example, this morning, we had green smoothies and scrambled eggs with tomatoes. For me, it's a great start to the day because I know that, after this kind of breakfast, our bodies are filled with healthy, beneficial nutrients. This means that during the day, it will be much easier to ignore the delicious fragrances of fresh baked pastries or the allure of potato chips on the store shelves.

3. **I buy bread, pasta, and potatoes once a month** and we eat them only when we really miss our childhood foods.

4. **I never skip breakfast** and I don't allow myself to get really hungry. I've noticed that if I don't eat in the morning because I'm in a rush, I keep grabbing tasty snacks for the rest of the day. In the evening, I feel tired and unhappy with myself for having eaten too much. So I firmly believe in breakfast and giving my body all the necessary building blocks with the first meal of the day.

SPECIAL FOODS

There are some special foods that I eat every day, not so much because I find them super delicious, but because, over the years, I've read so much about their benefits that I fell in love with them and put them on a pedestal. Here is a list of what I consider the most important foods to stay healthy—in order of priority.

1. **Wild berries.** When I eat them, I imagine how, over the summer, they nourished themselves with rich forest soil minerals and stored the best elements, which I can now give to my body.

2. **Farm eggs.** In my opinion, an egg is one of the most perfect foods. It stores high-quality building materials that can abundantly feed my cells.

3. **Bright green vegetables.** I mostly like leaf cabbage (kale), beet leaves, and broccoli. When I eat those vegetables, I feel satisfaction knowing that their color indicates their super rich and beneficial contents.

4. **Vegetables that grow in the ground, except for potatoes.** These are beets, carrots, and other root vegetables, which have the opportunity to live under the ground and collect its minerals.

5. **Oily fish.** You can find a lot of information about salmon and tuna. Some sources will praise their benefits, while others will emphasize the bad elements that can be found in them. Since it's almost impossible to know the truth, I choose to believe in the benefits of fish and wholeheartedly enjoy eating it. Of course, if it's possible, I choose wild caught fish, but I definitely don't turn my back on farm-raised salmon. I learned to love salmon while living in Los Angeles. After reading a book about the benefits of oily fish for the skin written by the dermatologist Dr. Nicholas Perricone, I made sure to bring fish home at least once a week.

6. **Avocados.** I fell in love with them thanks to one of my Mexican friends, who has the most perfect skin and hair, and who eats avocados daily.

7. **Nuts.** Nuts make it on my list because they are a perfect food. At least once every two weeks, I try to buy unroasted nuts, because during the roasting process they lose most of their best qualities. I prefer Macadamia and Brazil nuts because I was most impressed by their benefits when I was researching nutrition.

8. **Beef and chicken.** Every day we eat at least a small piece of meat. At one stage in my life, I went meat-free, but I didn't like the way I felt. The results of my blood work indicated that I had chosen a path that was not appropriate for my needs. I felt that my muscles lacked firmness, so I went back to eating meat. Vegetarians would probably say that I should buy supplements and eat more lentils and vegetables. But I know my body pretty well, and I know that they are not for me. I don't like the way legumes smell, their texture, or their effect on my digestive system. That's enough for me to say *no* and stick to meat.

Today my family and I appreciate meat. We don't eat a lot of it, but we are grateful for our strong and healthy bodies.

I sincerely believe in the food products I've just mentioned, and I try to integrate them in my family's daily meals. I can attest that this type of nutrition works because we hardly ever get sick or catch a cold. It shows that our immune system is strong and easily deals with bacteria and viruses.

Good seasonal food also makes the list of proper nutrition. For example, in Lithuania, a ripe plum or melon at the end of summer is more valuable than a peach or banana from the supermarket.

I am not a big fan of cereal. It seems lacking in vitality and vitamins, and is full of unnecessary carbs that quickly end up on my thighs. In the winter, however, when there are fewer fresh vegetables to choose from, I prepare porridge from whole-grain cereal. But I still consider it to be an average product.

I don't pay much attention to the remaining 30% of my food. I eat what I feel like eating because I know that my body can handle an occasional pastry, cracker, chocolate bar, piece of cake, or big cup of coffee. However, I try not to get carried away and keep a close eye on myself. If I order a piece of cake in a cafe, halfway through it, I usually feel that I've satisfied my craving, so I leave the rest of it on the plate. I do the same thing with potatoes or dishes that contain flour. I must admit that I find it a little difficult to stay away from rice crackers or wheat crackers, though. But, knowing myself, I buy smaller packages and don't eat them while watching TV or talking on the phone, because I know exactly what will happen—I'll overeat and disappoint myself.

Another simple rule is this: when cooking, I use very little seasoning. I picked up this habit on the cruise ships I mentioned earlier. I saw just how easy it was to get seduced by strong and stimulating tastes. That's how we lose self-control, overeat, and don't notice the feeling of satiation. Food, in my opinion, should be simple and easily prepared.

So my "70-30" rule works well. I don't have to think about food all the time, I don't feel like I am depriving myself, and I am content with my appearance and my weight. Before I sit down at the table, I ask myself whether the food on my plate will help me look and feel better, or whether it will lead me further away from my health goal and my desired appearance. When I answer this question, I know how much I can eat, and what my next dish is going to be. For example, recently we had a party. By the time it was over, I felt I had overeaten and was heavier. (It may not have helped that I had served whipped cream, but I'm not going to deprive myself.) I knew that if I put anything else in my mouth that day, it was going to be a piece of chicken or some blueberries.

THE SECOND HABIT:
WATCHING MY CARB INTAKE

Do you remember what I wrote about my ex-husband and his Atkins diet? That's when I saw with my own eyes how quickly excess weight can melt away when you give up carbohydrates.

Yes, it was difficult for him to eat only meat, cheese, and some vegetables, but the result was quick and obvious. There is no way I could follow the Atkins diet, but if you want to lose weight, certain aspects of this diet are worth adopting. Another diet that can teach you how to limit your carbs is the Keto diet.

Any nutritional plan can teach us something, but I don't recommend you follow them blindly and limit what you truly need, because long-term stress due to dieting may have negative consequences.

If you want to learn to regulate your weight, you need to understand what carbs are. I'm not going to give elaborate explanations. I'll just say that this food group includes baked goods, pasta, and potato dishes.

Fruit should also be included here. They belong to a slightly better category than bakery products, but if you want to lose weight, you should eat less fruit because it contains a lot of sugar. Vegetables are a great choice, but, when fighting extra pounds, stay away from the sweeter vegetables such as carrots, beets, or sweet potatoes.

Sugary drinks are also considered to be carbohydrates. In my opinion, we are just taking in more calories and sugar when we drink Coca-Cola, Sprite, and all of the other soft drinks overflowing on our store shelves.

Remember, *carbs are firewood that needs to be burned*. If there are too many carbs, they turn into fat and settle on our thighs, abdomen, and other areas of our bodies.

Just to be clear about how to reduce the amount of carbs and not feel stress, I'll give you an example from my own life. In the morning, I like to drink a fruit smoothie, but it contains a fair amount of sugar and carbs. If I substitute half of the fruit with vegetables, half of the carbs disappear, and I can still enjoy my morning dose of vitamins. Instead of the usual smoothie of bananas, strawberries, mangoes, plums, or any other seasonal fruit and berries, I have a more interesting version. I substitute mango with an apple, and banana with avocado. This way, I take in fewer carbs and get good fats from the avocado.

I have already told you about my habit of drinking my morning coffee with a piece of chocolate. However, on the days when I want to control my weight, instead of chocolate I have a piece of milk candy that satisfies my need for my morning ritual.

On days when I try to control my weight, I also don't eat my morning cereal. Instead, I have eggs with a fresh tomato salad and a small piece of bread.

I make similar substitutions during lunch. If, in the cafeteria, I eat my favorite beet soup, which is served with two boiled potatoes, I eat just one of them. And I completely ignore the potatoes that come with my main course. I eat only meat or fish with the vegetables.

The evenings are the hardest because I really want to snack. So it's important to have some protein snacks ready to go. In my fridge, I usually keep some meat, cheese (not the best choice, of course, but not the worst) and lots of cucumbers that I can dip in yogurt and enjoy. In my pantry, I have a few types of nuts and grains that help stave off the hunger, but I don't burden my body with excess carbs.

I eat like that only when I feel it's getting difficult to squeeze into my jeans. Or when I know that my body needs to take a rest from carbs because I had too many of them at a party.

THE THIRD HABIT:
PORTION SIZE

Now let's talk about portion sizes. Right now I like small portions. A couple of years ago, I was in a different stage of my life: I liked to have two full meals a day with generous portions, and yet not overeat. I was so tired of thinking about food that I decided to eat twice a day. I would brush my teeth in-between meals and just forget about food for the next 5 to 6 hours.

This method worked well at the time but not anymore. That's why I don't want to push my ideas on you and tell you how to eat. Only you know your needs and habits. If you don't like your weight, try experimenting with portion sizes, carb amounts, and find the best way to eat without creating stress for yourself or changing your lifestyle.

THE FOURTH HABIT:
A NEW ATTITUDE TOWARDS FOOD

Another important change took place when I established a relationship with food. A number of years ago, I didn't have a real connection with food—it was just a way to satisfy my hunger. When I became interested in psychology and energy, I wanted to learn where my food came from and what kind of energy it could provide.

I really love produce, especially if I purchase it at a market or if it comes directly from a farm.

I like the shapes and colors of tomatoes. I adore the aroma of some fruit, and it makes me happy to touch them and examine them. It really helps me not to overeat if I am grateful when I eat, and if I consciously put the food on my plate in my body. I never watch TV or sit at a computer and eat; if I direct my attention away from my food, I completely lose a sense of when to stop and often overeat.

Now people are becoming wiser and learning to eat differently. When we were under Soviet rule, we were happy when we had something to eat. Later, things changed, and we enjoyed the abundance we found on our store shelves. We stuffed ourselves with everything we could. Later we had to subject our bodies to diets, because we didn't like the extra kilos and how our appearance had changed.

Now people's relationship with food is calming down and is much more well-balanced. Intuitive eating, which, in my opinion, is the best and healthiest way to eat, is becoming increasingly popular. Unfortunately, there is one small problem. We can't eat intuitively if we don't know what our bodies are telling us, or worse still, we misread their signals.

For example, we may think that we want cookies, but that is a signal that our bodies need certain nutrients. If we had a closer relationship with food and each type of food that we eat, it would be much easier to trust our intuition. A while ago, it seemed to me that I craved potato dishes or hamburgers when I got hungry, but in reality, the scope of my menu was so poor that my body didn't know what other food it could wish for. So in order to eat intuitively, we need to have a friendly relationship with food and broaden the scope of our diet.

Now, while I am expecting my second daughter, I really worry about her being strong and healthy. So I focus my energy on healthy nutrition, and I am pleasantly surprised with my intuition.

During this pregnancy, I often go to the farm or the market and try not to react to the *callings* of pickles and pastries. I show my body that it has many other options.

What's interesting is that one month, I went to the market, saw a variety of produce, and knew exactly whether my body needed it or not. However, this approach works only with products that don't have a long list of ingredients or spices.

When I used to see strawberries, I could sense their sweetness, and I couldn't resist them. Their fragrance would follow me around all day until I gave in to the craving and ate as many of them as I wanted. Sometime later, I completely lost interest in berries—just looking at them left a sour taste in my mouth. Then I realized that I missed good oily fish. A similar story happened with cauliflower. For a month, my only breakfast was mashed cauliflower; I couldn't get enough of it. I almost never overate because my body, filled with vitamins and minerals, never craved cakes or hamburgers. What I understand now is that these cravings for specific *healthy* foods probably indicated that I was lacking some vitamin or essential nutrient, and my body knew *exactly* where to find it.

I don't want you to think that food should take up most of our time and attention. However, I can assure you that with some effort to eat better quality food, many of our problems will solve themselves. Good food and exercise improve not only our appearance but also our relationships.

Now with good nutrition, I have more energy, I don't have mood swings, and I feel more confident.

I don't even want to remember how I felt after indulging in pastry and cakes! How I would sit on a couch with no energy to do anything, and, instead of changing my eating habits, I would dump my anger and emotions on the people around me.

I still have an interest in food and try to preserve my relationship with it. And now, when I go to the market, I don't just look at the produce. I try to feel the energy of the person who grows it and sells it. I focus on the inner matters, which are invisible but felt with the heart.

WHERE TO START?

You have to start with tiny steps because our mind doesn't like big changes. I read an interesting book about forming habits and realized that it's very important to start with easy and simple steps. Then you have to repeat the desired action so that it becomes a habit that doesn't require much effort. If you want to learn to eat intuitively, you'll have to add variety to your diet. When you go to the market or the store, tell yourself to find some healthy food you wouldn't usually bring home. Of course, this means it can't be prepared or half-cooked. It's best if that product comes from the fruit, vegetable, or meat department. If you always shop in the supermarket, try to go to the farmers' market once a week and buy better quality food. If you eat three times a day while watching TV, try to eat once a day without being glued to some device.

You don't need to blindly trust me; try it for yourself. Then you'll see if it's worth continuing or not.

I have one more thing to say. If you don't change your actions, you'll have even more of what you have today. You can't keep living and eating the same way you have so far and expect different results. If you want to achieve anything, you have to change something. If you have an impulse to try something new while you are reading this book, go ahead and turn your new knowledge into action as soon as possible.

I swear by this statement: *I am what I allow inside me.* I am talking not only about food, but also about friends, everyday actions, movies, books, music, and many other things. I try to only allow inside of me the best I can find around me, and I stay away from anything that doesn't make me feel good or beautiful.

MY FIFTH HABIT:
THE MIRACLE OF EXERCISE

Last but not least, one of my daily habits is being outside and exercising. During my childhood, I loved exercising, but later I slowed down because it was so much more fun to *hang out* in cafes, watch movies, or spend time with my friends.

I thought that while I was young, I didn't really have to worry about working out. My body didn't look bad, so I didn't need to put in extra effort to keep it that way.

In Lithuania and other European countries where I worked as a model, gyms were not as popular as they are today. None of my friends worked out, so I had no particular motivation to exercise or practice a healthy lifestyle.

The benefits of exercise were perceived very differently in Los Angeles. This city has many sports clubs that are open 24/7. The media are full of pictures of celebrities working out with their personal trainers.

Los Angeles is full of hilly walking paths. It was common to get an invitation from a friend or a new acquaintance not only to have lunch but also walk their favorite route in the hills. Business or friendly conversations often happen while hiking in the surrounding mountains.

It's not hard to imagine that after about a year of living in California, I already knew the most beautiful paths in the hills and started to enjoy hiking.

I started going to the gym on the sad day when I saw the first signs of cellulite while trying on pants in the fitting room. I can't say that I enjoyed exercising, but eventually I got used to it, and active leisure became an integral part of my life. When I used to lose weight the old way, I hated exercise and workouts. Most of you probably know how excruciating it can be to run on a treadmill and wait for the desired number of calories to appear on the screen. After eating sweets, I felt guilty and would run to the gym on a full stomach to burn those 500 calories before they ended up on my thighs as fat or cellulite. I'm not proud of my attitude or lifestyle at the time, but I didn't know better. I just needed time, knowledge, and help to find inner peace and become friends with my body.

I have tried many types of sports and had countless trainers, who taught me how to achieve my desired results. Their beliefs were often very different from each other. Sometimes one trainer's opinion about how to eat and work out contradicted the opinion of another. At first it was confusing, but eventually I realized that there is no single truth, and nobody knows what's the best for my body.

I had to figure it out myself.

That's why I took a course at the National Sports Academy and decided to become a personal trainer myself. Most trainers tried to convince me that to get rid of cellulite, I had to lift heavy weights and grow muscles so that they would stretch my skin and eliminate the appearance of cellulite. I believed that for many years.

When heavy weights caused me knee pain, I discovered home workouts. I started to exercise for 20 minutes on a yoga mat and use my body weight as leverage. The lady who led the workout session on the internet often emphasized that if you wanted to have a nice backside, you have to move and warm up your muscles regularly. She recommended exercising without weights and moving muscles in different directions.

As I had no other option (my knees were in pain), I did those easy workouts 5 times a week. They would usually end up with stretching, for which I didn't have much time, but within a few months, I was pleasantly surprised to see my behind in the bathroom mirror. Who knew you could achieve such excellent results with workouts where you don't even break a sweat!?

This story teaches us that there is no single truth. We know our bodies better than

208

anyone else does. Workout plans and trainers may be helpful to get you going and understand the exercises. Later, when you know different types of sports and exercises, your workouts can be intuitive, same as eating.

Unfortunately, you can't start with your intuition. If you move very little and you don't know how your body may feel after one or another type of exercise, you won't get good intuitive advice from your body. First, you need to create an exercise list, and then you can expect that your body will hint at what it needs. So if you want to take the first step, do an activity that you have wanted to do for a while. If you are at least slightly drawn to something, it may be the most suitable place for you to start.

Sports have finally become an integral part of my life. I am not saying that I joyfully practice them every day, but finally, I don't feel the resistance I did before. On the days when I have healthy meals, go for a walk in the woods, and exercise, I feel like I'm on top of the world. I feel how my improved blood circulation carries vitamins and oxygen to my organs, and I am happy with what I see in the mirror.

I also want to share with you a little more about how I fell in love with nature and being outdoors. Until you realize how beneficial it is, it's difficult to find the time and will to do it. However, I have been convinced many times that there is always enough time for it. It's just a question of what we really want, what motivates us, and what our priorities are.

My main instructor in the Los Angeles beauty school was a very strict lady from Thailand. She kept telling us that if you don't like the outdoors, you won't have beautiful skin. She encouraged us to go to the mountains, parks, and forests. She personally loved the ocean the most.

This instructor insisted that beautiful skin requires good-quality oxygen. Only with good oxygen can your skin cells regenerate rapidly. She created a picture for us: as soon as your lungs are filled with fresh air, your cells start having a big party. They effectively multiply, clean up, get rid of toxins, and regenerate at a high speed. To make a long story short, when I enjoy the fresh air, my inner organs enjoy their party, and my skin is ecstatic. I never quite verified if this cell regeneration idea was 100 percent accurate, but I fully enjoyed this mysterious fresh air spa theory.

This instructor also taught me to look in the mirror before I got out of my car to go for a walk, and again after I had walked along the ocean. After spending time in nature, I always feel relaxed and rested, and I definitely look much better. It gives me energy and clears my brain.

Later, when I was exploring energy, I learned that nothing drains your energy in nature, (there are fewer people and other stimulants), so it's a perfect place to relax.

I try to be in the woods at least twice a week. And on some more difficult days, when I don't feel beautiful or emotionally stable, I make sure to find the time to walk outside almost every day.

If you don't already exercise regularly, and I managed to convince you that exercise and sports are important for your beauty and sense of well-being, try starting with small steps. Remember what I wrote about forming habits. Start with 5-minute exercises, but do them every day. It doesn't matter how long your workouts or walks are at first. It's only important that they be consistent, friendly to your body, and pleasant. You won't even notice how quickly you'll develop a new habit and enjoy the results.

Chapter ELEVEN

The invisible side of feminine beauty

I couldn't decide for the longest time how to start this chapter about inner feminine beauty. I think we can agree that this topic is a little intangible. Putting aside all mysticism and contemplation, we can look at some very simple things and draw some conclusions.

For many years, I found talks about one's inner glow really annoying. When I lived in Hollywood, we would talk about having a *good heart* or *inner beauty* somewhat jokingly or perhaps even cynically.

I met a lot of people who preached about inner values, but I never considered them to be a role model for me. I listened to their spiels politely but secretly waited impatiently for them to end.

I admired beautiful women who wore fashionable clothes and had the world at their feet. The ones who talked about inner beauty didn't look like that. Deep inside, I believed that any talk about inner beauty only came about when you couldn't begin to *dream* about outer beauty.

I can't blame myself, because the world around me kept reinforcing this belief. Los Angeles magazine covers featured women who knew how to pose and were drop-dead gorgeous.

Most of them were controversial personalities, but it didn't stop people from admiring them.

Rich men who came to Hollywood parties had long-legged girls in short cocktail dresses on their arms. Very few of them had any particular charisma or rich inner life.

My day-to-day life experience made me very sceptical: I believed what I saw. The reality was that, in my environment, there was not a single example that could convince me to strive for inner beauty.

The only inner quality all of the women worked for was self-confidence. A lot of *supposedly* smart people made a lot of *supposedly* smart statements that we would write down in our notebooks. For example, Marilyn Monroe is reported to have said, "A wise girl kisses but doesn't love, listens but doesn't believe, and leaves before she is left."

Self-confidence was that intangible quality you had to have, or at least fake. I couldn't quite understand what it was, and, at the time, I thought self-confidence was closely related to wearing designer clothes, living in luxury, and being full of arrogance, which comes across in your manners and facial expressions. All of the women I knew who were considered to be self-confident, could convincingly demonstrate their unattainability and uniqueness. They looked down on everyone as if wanting to emphasize that they belonged to a different category of people.

I was learning fast, and I often repeated my two favorite phrases: "*Self-confidence is true sexuality,*" and, "*Be the woman the man needs, but not the woman who needs him.*"

Thank God I was smart enough not to tattoo these statements on my body. The saddest part is that I believed these things not only when I lived in Hollywood, but for many more years afterwards when I returned from the United States to Lithuania.

The last time I wrote these sentences was about 6-7 years ago, which isn't that long ago. But I am happy to say that this attitude didn't stick with me for the rest of my life. With time, I managed to see the importance of inner beauty and I started developing it. Better late than never, right?

When I look back on my attitude, I realize that there was a gap I wasn't seeing. I just didn't see that the women I was learning from and whose images I wanted were *not happy*. They tried to pretend and convince the world that having men's attention and outer beauty opened all doors and brought happiness. But it simply wasn't true!

Not a single one of my girlfriends had an enviable relationship, and none of them felt happy. I don't understand how I was blind to that for so many years; I wasn't just an observer on the sidelines who watches the lives of beautiful women on a movie screen. I was behind the scenes, and I saw exactly what was going on. And yet I didn't.

A lot of the most beautiful women I have ever known cried on my shoulder because of men, loneliness, the inability to get out of toxic relationships, a dependence on pills, alcohol, and drugs. Many of them were hurting because of their husband's infidelity and hid it from society. They tried to numb their pain by shopping on Rodeo Drive.

Some changed their partners but still suffered because they just couldn't find love and fulfilling relationships. Each one's situation was unique, but none of them experienced joy and happiness.

So let's forget about Los Angeles' podiums and impressive parties around beautiful turquoise pools and turn to a more wholesome and perhaps spiritual environment where, among long skirts, incense, and Indian mantras, I was determined to discover my inner glow and true wisdom.

That was an excellent decision! To learn the truth and find out what kind of woman I wanted to become, I had to try another extreme.

For many years, I had a close friend I grew up with. As far back as I can remember, she was always close to me and part of my life. I have always loved her. Over the years, I have shared my life adventures with her. She became interested in the intricacies of women's inner life and self-discovery many years before I did.

Thanks to her, I managed to establish a bridge between two seemingly different worlds—the noisy and colorful world of Los Angeles and the quiet world of deep self-discovery. When I lived in California, we used to call each other about once a week. While sipping wine, I would tell her about my adventures with men, and she would tell me about her inner revelations.

After living in the United States for about 11 years, I returned to Lithuania. That's when I went through all kinds of inner crises, and it was very difficult to find inner peace. I had everything I needed for a picture-perfect life, but I wasn't happy.

Nothing was really missing: I was on my way to having a new and perfect life, where I would become a mother and feel fulfilled. I gave this new role a chance to make me happy, but a few years later, I realized that the miracle wouldn't happen. I had to stop looking for happiness outside of myself and, with some effort, start looking at the inner issues that prevented me from feeling happy with my life and myself.

I started attending seminars and exploring the inner life I didn't know or understand before. The first year, I basically pretended that I was in touch with my inner self and kept faking it. But every seminar, lecture, or meeting with a psychologist brought me closer to self-discovery; it's just that the changes were slower than I expected.

I've come to realize that understanding your inner life is not just about looking for peace, inner beauty, or harmony. It's also the business. There are many false teachers who fake their achievements. In this sense, things weren't very different from my life in Hollywood. Over there in Hollywood, girls and rich men faked their happiness while sitting in Ferraris, and over here, in the seminars, fake happiness was hidden under long skirts, white wraps, incense, and a whole bunch of nonsense I bought into over and over again, wasting as much money as I had on useless cosmetics. Los Angeles' beauties fool themselves into thinking that they are happy because they have material things others can only dream of. Spiritual teachers hide their lack of self-love behind melancholic gazes and never-ending talks about energy and their deep experiences, as well as their profound desire to make others happy.

For a while I did the same. I gravitated to the circle of new divas, talked to the forces of nature, connected with my ancestors, wished for fake happiness—until I got sick and tired of it all. Then I realized that life was too short to get stuck in one role or another.

Having said that, in this chaos I did manage to find something that gave me strength and self-confidence. I finally felt what it means to love yourself, at least a little, and be close to another person.

I also began discovering what it feels like to be at peace. Slowly, I began noticing a glow in my eyes that I rarely saw in other women, not because it's difficult to achieve, but because society and the media in general set us on the wrong path.

In the next part, we'll explore the real meaning of inner beauty. We'll discuss true inner glow and how to achieve it, and I'll tell you about my mistakes and discoveries. So, let's gets started!

What happens to a woman when she stops chasing outer beauty, drops the mask of a phony spirituality and devotion to others, and imagines that she has found some kind of middle ground ? I know, it sounds ironic, but after so much searching, I don't dare say that I understand anything or know the truth, or that I am ready to reveal new views of life.

What I can say, though, is that I would like to share my genuine life experience and sincere attitude towards life. While reading this, observe yourself and see which topics trigger certain emotions in you. Your sensations and feelings are the only true guide at the moment. If anything brings out your smile and admiration, it's probably something that touches your heart, and you can let it into your life. If you feel resistance, maybe you shouldn't go down this path just yet.

Words and stories have certain vibrations and energy: if something gives you pleasant sensations, it forms new paths in the invisible world, which will lead you to doing something good and beautiful for yourself. I always say that people who try to impose their ideas on you are just arrogant and self-important. So please, don't get caught up in their truths. Your life journey is unique. Only you know what you can do and what decisions you can make today.

217

WHAT MAKES A WOMAN UNATTRACTIVE?

The ugliest attitude that I can think of in a woman is clinging to people and manipulating them. We can be as beautiful as we want, but if we don't have anything to give anyone, and only want to suck everything out of them, it's not a good look.

I met many women I tried to socialize with, but no sooner had a friendship begun that I would find myself trapped in a web from which it was difficult to get out. They would force me to prove that I was a good friend, constantly demanding attention and the confirmation that I would be by their side if they needed me. I had to be devoted and ready to help. As soon as I started to live my life and didn't react to their needs, accusations would fly around. My so-called friends tried to make me feel guilty. I felt devastated after some of our conversations. I'm not blameless. I behaved the same way for many years myself. I used similar strategies with my husbands, friends, and other people close to me.

I didn't love myself and I didn't know how to find my place in the world, nor how to help myself. I had to constantly cling to people in order to feel important and needed. My husbands had to tell me thousands of times that they loved me. They had to keep proving in various ways that I was the most beautiful and the only one for them. And if, God forbid, they got tired and distanced themselves, I would make scenes, manipulate, and make them feel guilty for not appreciating my love and efforts.

If I had to draw a picture of myself, I'd draw a beautiful woman with a hungry parasite inside her that keeps looking for sources of energy to feed on. When someone finds themselves next to a woman like this, they have no choice but to get sucked into her drama and give away their precious life energy. Sometimes she manages to convince them that in return for their energy, she will give them love and attention, but after a while, it becomes harder to believe, and they just want to run screaming as far as they can get from her.

In reality, she's wounded, with many scars deep within her heart. She doesn't know how to make herself feel better, how to heal herself, so she clings to others as her only hope. The only way to be healed is to realize that anything you desire from others, you can give yourself, and then look for ways to deal with yourself and your needs.

Another quality that takes away from a woman's beauty and radiance is negativity.

I had a very beautiful friend for many years. We were close, but with time I grew tired of her. As soon as I saw her name on the phone, I knew that, in a few seconds, I'd find myself in a world of curses, complaints about men, gossip about other people, and dissatisfaction with life in general.

When I lived in a similar world, it didn't bother me. But as soon as I started working on my negative emotions, conversations with that friend seemed like a swamp I needed to avoid if I wanted to have a better quality of life.

Eventually, communication with that friend became impossible. I went to therapy sessions, learned not to judge others, started different meditation practices, and every day I tried to find something beautiful and positive to focus on. It took a lot of energy and effort to change my way of thinking. I had to let go of that friendship because it was impossible to nourish my inner life and feed on negative emotions at the same time.

While you are reading this part, think what kind of environment you create around you—with your words, behavior, and mood. It may seem insignificant at the moment, but over time, it becomes very important. Just think: your energy space is like your home. If you live like a slob, surrounded by dirty dishes, unpleasant odors, and a depressing mood, who will want to visit you? Maybe a wholesome and pleasant person will wander in by mistake, but they won't want to come back! A place like this attracts only those whose inner world is as negative and stinky as the environment into which he or she is invited.

After you read this part, ask yourself what the energy field surrounding you is like. Is it light, clear, easygoing, and pleasant? Or is it the opposite— dark and murky? Do your words, manners, attitudes, and conversation topics create a negative atmosphere, that no *light* person would want to approach?

The third attitude that takes away from your beauty is an exaggerated sense of self-importance.

Because we lack self-love and confidence, and don't have enough knowledge to deal with that, we decide to enhance our self-importance. Consciously or not, we put down others, judge them and tell ugly stories about them to make ourselves feel valuable and important. This shows just how desperate we are, and it's an unfortunate way to make oneself feel better. We need other people's love and support to feel beautiful and loved because we haven't learned to *love ourselves*. If we can't make sure that people next to us feel valuable and important, there's no point in hoping that they will appreciate our beauty and make us happy.

I remember how uncomfortable I felt around the men or women who talked non-stop about themselves, their admirable achievements, their extraordinary experiences, all the while showing no interest in me. I was used for one purpose only—to confirm their importance. Only after I realized how unpleasant it was to experience this, did I give up my own similar behavior and start to care about other people's well-being when they were around me.

I think we have discussed all the biggest enemies of beauty that may not always be physically visible but are certainly psychologically clear. All of our inner life shows up when we start communicating with others. We have to be alert and conscious if we want to create an environment that invites people to stay around us and makes us glow and express beauty and youthfulness.

If we manage to create a special atmosphere, people will love us and help us feel prettier and lovelier. Just think, isn't it nice to be around people who are positive and light? Next to them, the world becomes brighter, problems disappear, and everything seems possible and easy!

When people feel good around us, they look at us through a bright filter and see us as amazingly beautiful, magical, and unique. Isn't that what we want from our loved ones? I've seen it many times: when people feel happier and better when they are around us, they love and value us even more. And that provides us with another dose of beauty and glow!

A woman who is valued and happy is the most beautiful of all. Her eyes sparkle, and she goes through life with a radiant smile and contagious self-confidence.

THE END

AFTERWORD

I hope you enjoyed my book. For a long time, I dreamed of writing a book where I could share my knowledge and experience, but I mostly wanted this creation to be filled with advice about skin, nutrition, and inner values that could create a picture for you of how to become more beautiful than ever.

When I was writing this book, I was almost 43. I followed all the advice I have shared with you. For many years, I wandered around blindly in the maze because I wanted to feel better but didn't know how. I proved to myself that *the ship had not sailed* without me, and this is true for everyone. We can change the direction of our lives to any direction we choose. Sometimes we don't have enough knowledge or tools, but everything starts with a dream and a vision.

After all of these years, one of the most important lessons I learned is to be tolerant and forgiving towards ourselves. There are no mistakes, just life experiences. No matter what you do today, you can try and do better tomorrow. And with some extra effort, you can completely change your life and appearance in half a year.

When I was very young, I just wanted to be beautiful and have attention from men. Later, I wanted money and recognition. Later still, the time came for motherhood and inner order. That's when I realized that I had nothing in common with my husband, so I decided to get a divorce.

When it was just my daughter and me, a new man came into my life, and suddenly an even more interesting chapter began. I discovered my sexuality and found ways to convince myself that I could create a new relationship. It wasn't easy to go against my beliefs and the pressure from society. Now our relationship is so great, I could write a separate book just about that. As time goes by, our love is only getting stronger. However, this doesn't happen accidentally—we both devote a lot of time and attention to it.

Now, as I am finishing up this book, there is another little heart beating inside my body. After eight years of living together, we are going to have a little daughter before my 43rd birthday, and I'll become a mother again. I can't wait to see my little girl and welcome her into our wonderful, loving family.

I am not sure if I want to have more children. All I know is that I would never say *no* to myself and create unnecessary doubts in my head that could stand in the way of achieving my dreams. And I have a lot of dreams! Someday I would like to write a book about relationships and feminine sexuality.

I also dream about having my own line of skin care products, where all the facial products would be perfect and effective, and you wouldn't have to waste time and money finding a way to take care of your skin.

I refuse to believe that as a woman ages, her appearance, her sense of well-being, and her sexual life go downhill. I am deeply convinced that all those things depend on our beliefs and attitudes towards ourselves. I can honestly state that at 42 I feel happier and more beautiful than I did at 20.

I know that as long as I have this philosophy and discipline, everything will be ok. I hope not to get overly attached to any beliefs because I know I'll be able to quickly change my attitude and behavior as needed. This attitude helps me go forward and feel like a free woman who can create a beautiful life and choose her own direction. I've come a long way, and I hope you will too. That's what I sincerely wish for you.

If today your life and your body don't look the way you want them to, don't give up! Don't think that it's impossible to change. It's just a sign that you haven't had the knowledge or the inner resources that could help you. Now you have much more information to rely on than before you started reading this book, and chances are better than ever that you will fulfill your dreams!

Good luck!

Ruta

BE LIKE A FLASHLIGHT:

No matter in which direction you are pointed,
you shed light.
Everything depends on attitude, and
external circumstances are not very important.

RUTA BANIONYTE

.

Printed in Great Britain
by Amazon